Wood
Becomes
Water

Chinese Medicine in
Everyday Life

20th Anniversary Edition

Wood Becomes Water

Chinese Medicine in Everyday Life

Gail Reichstein

New Forewords by
Robert Rex
Jessica DePete, L.Ac., M.S.
Florence Patsy Roth, L.Ac., M.S.

Illustrated by Pat Tan and Marie T. Keller

KODANSHA USA, INC.

Kodansha USA, Inc.
451 Park Avenue South, New York, NY 10016, U.S.A.

Distributed in the United Kingdom and continental
Europe by Kodansha Europe Ltd.

This book is not intended as a substitute for medical
advice from physicians. The reader should regularly
consult a physician in matters relating to their health
and particularly in respect to any symptoms that may
require diagnosis or medical attention.

Published in 2018 by Kodansha USA, Inc.

Library of Congress has cataloged the earlier edition as
follows:

Reichstein, Gail.
Wood becomes water: Chinese medicine in everyday
     life/by Gail Reichstein; illustrated by Pat Tan.

   p.   cm.
   Includes bibliographical references and
   index.

1. Medicine, Chinese.   I. Title.
R601.R335   1998
610'.951—dc 21   97-31947

ISBN-13: 978-1-56836-588-6

Book design by Pat Tan
Cover design by Tomoe Tsutsumi

Manufactured in the United States of America on
     acid-free paper

21 20 19 18   5 4 3 2 1

CONTENTS

FOREWORD

In the twenty years since *Wood Becomes Water* was first published, my wife Gail Reichstein received many wonderful and heartfelt letters from readers and people familiar with her work as an acupuncturist and teacher. In response to one of these notes, an inquiry about the significance of the title, Gail wrote:

> "Essentially, the title is meant to evoke the entirety of the Sheng cycle -- from Wood to Fire to Earth to Metal to Water. Though I know it is sometimes confusing for people, I chose this wording because I loved the poetry of it; both the sound of the words and the image of the energy moving from element to element."

Gail treated each communication she received as if it were from the reader of the very first copy she ever sold. Every one, every question, every comment mattered. In fact, this is how she lived her life—every one, every word, every element matters.

During my twelve-year marriage to Gail, she always sought the magic—the magic of herbs, the magic of healing, the magic of calling in her partner, the magic of calling in and attending to our child, and the magic of being called to her next purpose. Together, we marveled at the magic that could be found everywhere, whether in her favorite books, in herbs we found in our gardens and lawn, in the things our son told us. She lived her life with magic as her guiding force: live for what is—the now that brings joy, beauty, abundance, love; not for scarcities that aren't.

In thinking about how to revise and update her influential book, Gail wrote:

> "After more than twenty years of experience as an acupuncturist and writer, I have found that this book has remained relevant and important to those readers who seek information about the theory and practice of Chinese Medicine. There are few books on

the market that cover even a portion of this information, and I want to be sure to maintain my book's unique place in the literature. As an accessible introduction to the theories and concepts of Chinese Medicine, *Wood Becomes Water* properly belongs among classic foundational texts like *The Web That Has No Weaver* and *Between Heaven and Earth*."

Unfortunately, her intention to update *Wood Becomes Water* didn't go as planned. She died, suddenly, in August of 2016. Instead of being able to incorporate the new insights that Gail was ruminating on, we are left with what she originally wrote, which continues to be amazing, illuminating, and timeless. Gail constantly pushed herself (and her clients, at times) into learning about our bodies from the inside and the outside. Her clinical treatments, as well as her words, allowed her clients and her readers to heal in unexpected ways. In attending to the magic of the elements (as they relate to the seasons on Earth), as well as the ebbs and flows within our bodies, Gail left us with powerful teachings for self-healing and self-awareness.

A few years ago, Gail received the following note from a reader:

> "I am taking the liberty of contacting you to express my gratitude for having shared *Wood Becomes Water*. The book has inspired me beyond words. I am a yoga teacher and teach Yin Yoga amongst other styles. Before most of my classes, I will reread passages or chapters of your book. I always seem to find something new and inspiring."

We can never understand the reasons why someone has left us. Perhaps, we'll understand when we join them, later. But for now, we're not meant to (a) join them, or (b) understand why right now. We can pray and meditate in hopes of helping our departed loved ones achieve whatever they are meant to achieve on other planes. We can have visitations (through dreams, clairvoyant experiences, etc.) that can obtusely explain the what's and the why's. But most importantly, for us still on this plane, we can incorporate their essence, their compassion, their teachings into our lives to help make this realm more tolerable for us, our relations, those less fortunate, and build (re-build) our personal universe—our lives—with joy, beauty, and love.

Robert Rex
2018

FOREWORD

It is not hyperbolic to say that Gail Reichstein gave me my life back. Not only did she help me heal when all else failed; she also gave me the gift of Chinese medicine, which has become my life's work.

When I met Gail, I was a twenty-four-year-old woman who felt and functioned like an eighty-four-year-old. A year prior to our first acupuncture session, I woke up one morning to find that my body had seemingly turned against me. Every joint felt rusted closed, every muscle ached. Lymph nodes swelled and fever flared. "I must have the flu," I thought at the time, not knowing that these symptoms would last far longer than a week. Over the next few months, I watched my hands turn into my grandmother's hands – gnarled, swollen, stiff and sore. My right elbow locked at a 45-degree angle, and protested loudly when I, out of habit, extended my arm to open a door or reach for my shampoo in the shower. Color had drained from my face, I lost weight without trying, and I barely had the energy to start a day, let alone finish one. I became anxious and depressed.

During this time, I saw a host of doctors – general practitioners, rheumatologists, infectious disease specialists, and Lyme specialists. I was diagnosed with Lyme, bebesia, erlichiosis by some; with fibromyalgia by another; rheumatoid arthritis by several; and not-quite-lupus by others. I was given antibiotics, anti-malarials, and antidepressants. Anti, anti, anti. And nothing improved.

As anyone who has managed a chronic illness can attest to, being sick invites a lot of suggestions from people who want to see you get better. Realizing that medications were not helping me, but unfamiliar with alternative and traditional medical approaches, I followed every lead that came my way. I went to a chiropractor. I received light therapy and craniosacral therapy and reiki. I eliminated dairy and wheat and hundreds of other foods from my already-vegetarian diet based on kinesiological testing. I started meditating. I found a good psychotherapist. All of these practices helped, but nothing came close to resolving my issues.

One of the things that gave me the most relief was Qigong. I found a teacher after reading that this Chinese practice was useful for chronic pain and the idea of moving energy through the body resonated with me. And yet, when Gail's phone number was given to me by a neighbor who had experienced symptoms similar to mine, I stashed it in my overflowing health folder without giving it much thought. I felt thin-skinned and vulnerable and the idea of needles in my body felt threatening.

When I finally reached out to Gail, I was feeling close to hopeless. I still remember filling out her intake forms and circling every joint in angry red pencil to show her where my pain was. I walked into her office feeling ready to be disappointed, as I'd been so many times before. And then she came out to greet me.

Gail was warm, and kind, and gentle, and knowledgeable. She looked at me through a lens so different from every other lens I'd been seen through before. And she became my partner in healing.

Over the next year, with Gail's caring guidance, I grappled my way out of the worst depths of my illness. The year after that, I regained strength and resilience. And in the year after that, I was able once again to look to the future. At Gail's suggestion, I enrolled at her alma mater, the TriState College of Acupuncture, to study the art, philosophy, and practice of Chinese medicine.

After three years of school and thirteen years of private practice, I remain awed by the effectiveness of this medicine. Like Gail, I am not a Five Elements practitioner, yet the Five Elements inform my interactions with each and every client. Take Brian, a sinewy young man who was tightly-coiled, ready for action, easily frustrated by anything that obstructed his plans. Brian came to me for bordering-on-painful tension in his upper back, neck and shoulders. To be effective, my interactions with Brian needed to acknowledge his Wood excess – he needed the space to uncoil but also a clear vision of what was to come. Points such as Liver-3 and Liver-14 were always incorporated into Brian's treatments, and were also prescribed for self-acupressure at home. With regular treatment, self-care, stress-reduction and flexibility exercises, Brian learned to manage his constitutional inclination towards a Wood imbalance.

Or take Martha. Martha carried her weight in her belly and hips, and almost glowed the color yellow, the color of the Earth element. Her greatest need was to be understood by others and she gave selflessly to those she cared about, even to her own detriment. Her body ached in damp weather, and when she was upset, she experienced digestive disturbances. In my interactions with Martha, I kept in mind that to feel safe and secure, Martha needed to feel heard and supported. Her acupuncture treatment and home acupressure treatment always included Spleen-6, Spleen-9 and Stomach-36, the most powerful points for regulating the Earth element.

Elizabeth's husband had passed away four years ago. She carried on but was still deeply grieving and was often overtaken by sadness. When she first began treatment with me, I could hear her inability to fill her lungs as she spoke, and the skin around her eyes was devoid of color, almost translucent. She had become extremely susceptible to colds and her reason for starting treatment was to strengthen her immune system. Elizabeth's Metal element was out of balance due to the tragic loss of her husband. With repeated treatments including Lung-1 and Lung-3, her crying jags became less frequent and she found herself more able to smile.

Like Gail, I love practicing a medicine that acknowledges our constitutional tendencies, our lifestyles, habits, preferences, and patterns. I loved working with Brian, Martha, and Elizabeth, and meeting each of them wherever they needed to be met to do their deepest healing, as Gail did with me when I was at my lowest. As she asked in her author's note, "What kind of medicine could possibly care whether I liked evenings or mornings better?" Each client is a mystery, unique and yet part of a greater cosmological pattern, and every habit, every symptom, every word, even the very sound of his or her voice, is a clue that helps their practitioner support their healing.

Before starting school, I ordered Gail's book and was unsurprised to read in her author's note that her relationship with acupuncture began much as my own had. That same dogeared volume sits beside me as I write this, and I think there are more sentences highlighted in yellow than not -- lasting evidence of a novice's zeal for her mentor's wisdom. It is the book I revisit for inspiration and the book I give to clients who want to deepen their understanding of Chinese medicine. And now, it is the book I tenderly peruse when I want to hear the voice of my healer, my inspiration, and my mentor. May this book, and your relationship with Chinese medicine either as patient or practitioner, serve you well, in body, mind, and spirit.

Jessica DePete, L.Ac., M.S.
2018

FOREWORD

Since Gail Reichstien wrote *Wood Becomes Water: Chinese Medicine in Everyday Life* two decades ago, alternative medicine has gone through a revolution of sorts. Once considered way out of mainstream medical practice, acupuncture shingles can now be found across America, sometimes in the smallest towns. Yoga has become widely recognized as an effective technique to help combat everything from stress and anxiety to osteoporosis. Herbal remedies that were once available only in the Chinatowns of American cities can now be found in local pharmacies. Many alternative therapies are even covered by standard health insurance policies.

In reality, there is nothing "alternative" about Chinese medicine; its methods have been around for thousands of years. It is only in relatively recent history that treating the problem, rather than the whole person, has become the norm. Slowly and reluctantly, Western medical practitioners are coming to accept the fact that people do not experience their bodies, minds, and spirits as separate entities, but as one, integrated whole. To heal the body, one must look both inside and outside it.

The Five Element theory encompasses all the ways we exist in the world and the ways in which the world exists in us. In order to be healthy individuals, we must live in harmony with the world around us. Gail's book serves as a Five Element primer, helping us to understand how we experience the elements in our daily lives on the earth, and what we can do to bring ourselves into harmony with these elements.

Today, as we grapple with the current climate change crisis, this book becomes more important than ever. Nothing illustrates the connection between the body and the earth better than the Five Element cycle; when the elements are in balance, the body is in balance, and the earth is in balance. As she explains so beautifully in her conclusion, "We suffer the same illnesses, and will heal from the same cures. We are that closely intertwined."

Gail Reichstein was an inspiration to me as a healer. Through this new edition of her book, her inspiration will reach farther and wider. Gail understood the heartbeat of the earth and imparts to us in these chapters many of the ways the Five Elements resonate with us.

Florence Patsy Roth, L.Ac., M.S.
2018

AUTHOR'S NOTE

When people learn that I'm an acupuncturist, their first response is often "Oh . . . how did you decide to go into *that*?" The note of puzzlement in their voices is unmistakable. What I really hear them asking is "Are you for real? Is there something worthwhile in this Chinese medicine stuff?"

The answer is yes, but I usually start by telling them "It was a journey." That seems the only way to describe how I moved from the accepted worldview of my parents and teachers into the holistic universe that governs so many Eastern arts, Chinese medicine among them.

It was a journey that began in my early twenties, when I was seeking relief from pain in my joints that had bothered me since childhood. What had been ambiguously diagnosed as "growing pains" and "maybe arthritis" had taken a turn for the worse, and I worried about becoming seriously disabled. So when a friend told me that acupuncture had helped his mother's arthritis, I decided to try it.

I'd had no idea what to expect from acupuncture, but I was blown away on the first visit: It felt *good*, and it was different from anything I had ever known. Not only that, the questions I was asked during treatment also generated a strange excitement in me: They were so unlike anything any doctor had cared about before. Which season did I like best, and which one did I like least? What kind of foods did I eat? Did I crave sweet flavors or salty? Sour or bitter? At what time of day was my pain worse or better? Was I happy with my living situation? What exactly did my pain feel like, and what part of which joints did it affect?

At first it was a game, answering so many questions about myself. But slowly it dawned on me that this acupuncturist was not asking questions out of mere politeness—she was, in fact, drawing information from my answers. She really wanted to know that I liked broccoli but hated mushrooms, and that the ache before rain was heavy and diffuse, whereas the pain before snow was like knives. I wondered what this information could mean to her. What kind of medicine could possibly care whether I liked evenings or mornings better?

When the acupuncturist recommended that I stay away from sugar and alcohol because they caused "dampness," I agreed to try. I had no idea what dampness was or why it might be bad for my joints, but I was willing to experiment. In fact, it was a relief to find something I could do to help myself.

Over the next weeks and months I learned that "dampness" did make my joint pain worse, and that avoiding dampness-causing factors made it better. As I learned how to control dampness in my life, my joints improved, my energy level increased, and my concentration and mood got better. But even more exciting was the revolution in my thinking—I suddenly understood that my actions would affect my health. Whereas I'd always thought disease was random—I caught a cold, or developed arthritis, or had good and bad days for no apparent reason—I was beginning to see that my health was strongly influenced by what I did, saw, ate, felt, etc., on a daily basis.

My eating habits were the first to change as I discovered how various foods affected not only my joints but everything about me—my weight, my sense of well-being, the light in my eyes, etc. But there were other changes, too, like the day I complained about anxiety and heart palpitations—was there anything I could eat to help that? My acupuncturist calmly replied that I could first of all stop wearing red shirts like the one I had on that day. I laughed. How could the color of my shirt make a difference?

She took my skepticism in stride and explained that the color red was "connected to" my heart through the element of Fire. Like Fire, the color red would heat me up and stimulate my system. As anxiety and palpitations were symptoms (in my case) of overexcitement, more stimulation in the form of the color red was not what I needed.

So began my journey into Chinese medicine, and the Five Element cycle that is one of its foundations. Fire was joined by Wood, Earth, Metal, and Water, and in the following years I not only healed from my joint pain, I healed a whole life's worth of disconnection from my body, environment, feelings, and food. In time, these Five Elements—which had once seemed a quaint construction—took on an intelligence and enormous beauty that I had previously failed to recognize.

Using imagery and symbolism, the Five Elements linked physical ailments with emotions, behaviors, and also with the forces of nature—with weather, color, sound, time, space, and more. I began to recognize my universe as a symphony composed of these five themes, repeated in endless variations. Appearing all around me, the Five Elements showed me order where I had previously seen only chaos, and connected my body and soul to a world from which I had once felt cut off.

To this day I am amazed at the power of Chinese medicine to effect sophisticated cures that are described in such simple terms. The language of Wood, Fire, Earth, Metal, and Water is powerful *because* it is not scientific; rather it is a symbolic language that evokes images more than single events or anatomical parts. It is a language of poetry, and the practice of Chinese medicine is a poetic art with its own cadence, power, and infinite interpretations.

The upshot of it all is that what you wear will affect your migraines and your irritable bowel; what you eat and what you look at on a day-to-day basis will affect your relationships, your emotions, and your physical being. These are not new ideas, but putting them into action can require a leap of faith: It's one thing to agree that "everything is connected," but quite another to treat your headaches by rearranging your furniture, or to improve your allergies by changing your diet in the spring. Such behavior seems irrational because we can't imagine a plausible connection between our homes and our headaches, sugar and our immune systems, or our bodies and the body of the Earth.

The genius of Chinese medicine is that it establishes these connections in clear and consistent ways. It provides theories that clarify our relationships (with food, seasons, emotions, etc.) and practices that create healing by strengthening those relationships. In defining our health and healing so broadly, Chinese Medicine challenges our notions of what "medicine" can be; over the years I have learned to love its expanded vision, and this book is my attempt to share it. An exploration of what excites me most about Chinese medicine, the book includes images (snapshots, perhaps) of a worldview that is whole. I hope it will encourage readers to see their lives and their surroundings in a fuller context, that they may be inspired to participate in the healing of themselves, their loved ones, and the Earth, our holiest mother.

ACKNOWLEDGMENTS

My first thanks go to the Tri-State Institute of Traditional Chinese Acupuncture, which taught me how to do what I love and gave me the freedom to do it in a creative and joyful way. To Mark Seem, the institute's founder and director, I am deeply grateful for having shown me the way to my own healing, my life's work, and my greatest teacher. I also give thanks to my other acupuncturists: Carolyn Bengston, Beverly Bakken, and Dan Plovanich.

I am grateful to my encouraging readers—Sarah Schenck, Mo Ogrodnick, Margaret Loftus, Lawrence Reilly, Maureen Graney, Lorie Dechar, Melissa Padovani, Jean Railla, and Mark Seem; they helped to form this book and their excitement for it kept me going. And especially to Sarah Durham, whose constant friendship and perfect sense of structure have helped me through countless difficulties in this endeavor and so many others. Thanks also to my clients, some of whose stories appear in this book; I am truly grateful for the chance they have given me to learn and to teach. To Deborah Baker, my editor, who kept me grounded throughout the writing of this book; to Pat Tan, who gave it her graceful designs and illustrations; and to everyone at Kodansha who had a hand in its production.

Special blessings to my parents, Ronald and Toby Reichstein, and to my whole wonderful family, whose continuous love and support have been a source of profound strength. To my agent, Maureen Graney, who was truly a midwife for this project, and whose rock-steady advice, generosity, and enthusiasm brought it to life.

And finally, deepest gratitude to my friend and mentor, Llorraine Neithardt, who has spent lifetimes teaching me how to meet my destiny with love and integrity. Without her none of this would have been possible.

To all of those who have contributed to this book, and to the Great Spirit who contributes to everything, I extend my heartfelt thanks and deepest honor.

INTRODUCTION

The four practices addressed in this book—acupuncture, QiGong, dietary therapy, and Feng Shui—compose a significant portion of Chinese healing arts. (Other practices, including herbology, astrology and the *I-Ching*, properly belong in the category as well, although they are not explored in this volume.) While these disciplines are entire arts unto themselves, together they constitute a worldview that unifies theory and practice in a way few other cultures have equaled.

Many books are available that introduce readers to the fundamentals of each of these disciplines, and this book does not retread that ground. Instead, it views each practice through the lens of the Five Element system, highlighting those parts of it that reflect Five Element principles. In the case of acupuncture and dietary therapy, I have drawn upon long-standing Five Element traditions; with QiGong and Feng Shui, however, there are fewer such interpretations available, and I have taken some liberties in order to view them from a Five Element perspective. This book thus presents a partial exploration of several vast disciplines; it is by no means intended to be a comprehensive education or a manual for treatment of serious illness. Readers are encouraged to obtain professional advice about their health conditions, and to pursue further information on any topics that are of interest. For this purpose there is a reference section at the end of the book.

The following brief orientations are provided for readers who are unfamiliar with the basic theories of Chinese medicine, Feng Shui, and QiGong. They contain certain concepts and vocabulary that are referred to throughout the book. Those who already understand the basics of these disciplines may prefer to skip these sections and continue on to the next chapter.

QI

Central to all disciplines of Chinese healing is the universal energy known as qi (pronounced "chee"). Qi animates life and growth, powers movement, and effects change. It is very similar to the modern scientific notion of energy—the capacity of a system to do work. In science, energy is studied in electric, magnetic, atomic, chemical, mechanical, thermal, potential, and kinetic forms, among others. Qi is similarly known in China as "heat qi," "electrical qi," "weather qi," etc., and within the body as "air qi," "food qi," "upright qi," and so on. Qi is energy, and it remains the same whether it occurs in a rainstorm, an electrical system, or the kidneys, just as the electricity used to light a bulb is the same whether it is generated by magnets, chemicals, atomic fusion, or a water wheel; the underlying force expresses itself in a variety of ways.

According to the Taoist cosmology that is one of the fundaments of Chinese medicine, qi exists in the heavens, on earth, and in the human body. In the heavens it creates weather, moves the planets along their orbits, and animates all living things. It governs the relationship between Yin and Yang, the processes of waxing and waning, and the courses of evolution and development. On earth, qi is present wherever there is energy. It gives organisms the power to move and metabolize, and creates heat, electricity, magnetism, etc. It creates power, fuel, and the passage of time, and is the ruler of prosperity and decline.

In the body, qi is energy and movement, and the activator of all bodily transformations. It is like the electricity that runs through a lightbulb in order to make it work. Qi is present everywhere in the body, but its daily creation relies on the food we eat and the air we breathe. The ancient pictogram for qi showed the vapor steaming up from a bowl of cooked rice; it thus has connotations with both food and air, though it is not exactly like either of them.

Qi has been variously translated as "energy, " "vapors," and "breaths," and all of these definitions appropriately imply a kind of motive force. This force is the energy of life, and a primary factor in the health and prosperity of all living things. Over centuries, observations of qi and its movements gave rise to many different practices, whose aim it was to enhance and regulate qi flow. Some of these practices, like acupuncture and QiGong, focused on the microcosmic qi of the human body, while others, like Feng Shui and astrology, emphasized the macrocosm. Each practice developed myriad strategies for evaluating and affecting qi flow, understanding that to harness the power of healthy energy was to live a fuller, healthier, and more satisfying life.

ACUPUNCTURE

Acupuncture is believed to have begun around the third millennium B.C.E.* Shells and bones from that period that are inscribed with Chinese characters show how herbs and stone needles were used to stimulate certain points on the body.

In acupuncture, the body is viewed as a system of interconnected *organs* and *meridians,* through which qi flows to power body function and maintain health; disruptions in qi flow cause symptoms and create illness.

Organs, as they are understood in Chinese medicine, are different from their Western anatomical counterparts. They describe certain energy centers, and specific functions that derive from those centers, but they *do not* describe the health or function of their related anatomical organs, except in some cases. This is important to remember, because an imbalance in the Chinese Spleen or Liver, for instance (distinguished in this text by an initial uppercase letter), will most likely not correlate to any medical problem in the Western spleen or liver. It may be easiest to think of Chinese organs as sort of doubles of the Western ones—existing alongside them, often changing in response to them, but as having functions that are distinct and independent.

There are twelve main organs—the Lung, the Large Intestine, the Stomach, the Spleen, the Heart, the Small Intestine, the Bladder, the Kidneys, the Heart Protector, the Triple Heater, the Gallbladder, and the Liver.

Each organ has specific functions, which are detailed in the following chapters.

* B.C.E. refers to "before Christian Era," and its counterpart, C.E., refers to the current Christian Era.

The Spleen, for instance, is said to control qi, build blood, and transform and transport food, among other things, while the Lungs disperse fluids, rule the surface of the body, and circulate qi in the chest.

Together, the organs accomplish all of the body's functions, like digestion, breathing, cell repair, muscle movement, and so on. In part, they do this by moving energy and fluids around the body so they can undergo the necessary transformations at appropriate times and places. Sometimes qi needs to be sent downward in the body—from Stomach to Small Intestine during digestion, for instance, or from Lungs to Kidneys during breathing. At other times qi may need to be directed upward, outward, or inward. Such movements are variously described in Chinese medicine as descending, ascending, dispersing, and consolidating movements. They are an important part of physical health and key indicators of organ function.

The twelve organs are grouped in pairs, with each pair corresponding to one of the Five Elements. The Lung and Large Intestine correspond to Metal, for example, while the Heart and Small Intestine correspond to Fire. (Another organ pair, the Heart Protector and Triple Heater, also corresponds to Fire, which is the only element to have two organ pairs.)

The organs are connected to *meridians*—channels that link the organs and distribute their energy throughout the body. There are twelve main meridians, named for and connected to each of the twelve major organs. These meridians carry the same Five Element correspondences as the organs whose names they share. In addition, there are fifty-nine other channels that distribute qi to other areas of the body. But whereas organs work deep inside the body, meridians are closer to the surface, where they are accessible to touch, acupuncture needling, and a variety of other techniques.

When the organs or meridians don't function properly, symptoms will arise. Depending on what they are and where they occur, symptoms reveal which organs and meridians are unhealthy. Headaches along the sides of the head, for instance, indicate Gallbladder dysfunction—either in the meridian or the organ itself, or both. Belching, on the other hand, indicates a particular kind of

Stomach imbalance, in which the Stomach can't descend its qi, which rises up into the throat instead of descending.

Problems of the organs and meridians—and the symptoms that reveal them—are treated at certain acupuncture *points* on the skin, which are junctures where the energy of the meridian and its corresponding organ are accessible. At these points, acupuncturists use needles, heat, and other techniques to rectify imbalances in body energy. Energy can be strengthened or *tonified* when it is weak, or *dispersed* when it is stagnant.

DIETARY THERAPY

Dietary and herbal therapies are common in China and gaining popularity in the West. They treat bodily illnesses by using food and herbs as medicines. The flavor, color, shape, and thermal nature of individual foods determine the manner in which they will affect body energy—in Chinese medical terms, whether they raise or lower qi, for instance, or increase Lung Yin, and so on; together these qualities compose the *energetic* nature of every food.

This book explores the energetics of certain groups of foods as they accord with the Five Element system. The food qualities discussed include Flavor, Thermal Nature, Shape, and Color.

> **Flavor.** In a classical work compiled between the second century
> B.C.E. and the seventh century C.E., five "flavors" were determined
> to correspond with each of the Five Elements. The five flavors
> were sour, bitter, sweet, pungent, and salty. Every food is aligned
> with one or more of these flavors, and every flavor has specific
> effects on body energy. The pungent flavor, for instance, disperses
> energy, while the bitter flavor cools it and directs it downward
> (toward the eliminatory organs).

Thermal nature. In addition to its flavor, every food has a thermal aspect, which describes whether it cools or warms the body, or has a neutral effect. Thermal nature does not refer to measurable temperature but to energetic qualities that are classified as cold or hot.

Shape. The shape or growth pattern of fruits, vegetables, and grains is also considered an important energetic indicator by some practitioners. Foods that grow upward on strong stems and stalks—like asparagus and wheat, for instance, raise body energies upward (toward the chest and head), while foods that grow in layers—like cabbage and onions—are generally strengthening.

Color. Colors, in general, have long-standing Five Element correspondences, and food colors accord with them.

There are many discrepancies within the field of dietary therapy about the energetics of particular foods. Some authors classify coffee as warming, for instance, while others call it cooling. Nearly every food is interpreted in more than one way by more than one author, so dietary therapy can vary from practitioner to practitioner. Readers are not only encouraged to use good reference books, but also to learn to use their own judgment and interpretive powers. Please note that the particulars of herbal therapy are not included in this volume as they are best pursued under the supervision of a qualified herbalist.

QIGONG

QiGong refers to the cultivation and preservation of qi. It literally means "energy work that requires a lot of time and effort," * and is a combination of movement, meditation, breathwork, and self-discipline that cultivates the health of the mind-body-spirit. As a forerunner of and companion to the martial arts, QiGong also reinforces physical power. Historically, there are references to the cultivation of qi and the training of the breath in the *I-Ching,* which is four thousand years old; like many practices, however, QiGong was not formally named and systematized until much later.

QiGong consists of both physical and metaphysical exercises. While it recognizes the organs and meridians of Chinese medicine, QiGong's metaphysical focus views the human body within the larger context of the cosmos; it seeks to establish harmony between heaven, earth, and humanity. Thus QiGong is concerned with those human attributes that link us to both heaven and earth, defining them as Three Treasures—Energy, Essence, and Spirit. Energy is qi, the motive force of the universe. Essence is more like its soul—the substance and the meaning of all that exists. Spirit comprises mind and awareness. Each of these Three Treasures exists in heaven, on earth, and within the human body, connecting them together functionally and materially.

The various practices of QiGong are intended to strengthen and regulate the Three Treasures, and thereby to promote harmony in the universe. Breathing exercises help to build and regulate Energy and Spirit; meditation regulates the Spirit, while physical exercises promote both Energy and Essence. Proper lifestyle also helps to preserve Essence and calm the Spirit. Together, these practices are considered key to health and longevity.

QiGong's physical exercises fall into two broad categories, called *internal* and *external* exercises. External exercises work primarily with the four limbs. They tone and regulate the body's muscles and flesh, and help to build qi. External exercises are considered the basic tools of health and longevity, and are fundamental to any QiGong practice. Internal exercises work with the internal organs and with the body's Essence and Spirit. Rather than contributing to health and longevity only, internal exercises also involve spiritual training and the quest for enlightenment.

While QiGong masters often serve as healers for others, most people use

* Yang Jwing-Ming, *The Root of Chinese Chi Kung.*

QiGong as a personal practice that helps them to maintain health, fitness, and peace of mind. For many it is also a tool of spiritual growth, cultivating harmony with the universe and bringing wisdom, power, and heightened sensory capabilities. This book introduces some basic QiGong exercises, meditation techniques, and breathing practices.

FENG SHUI

Feng Shui, which means "Wind, Water," concerns itself with the way energy flows through space—through indoor spaces like houses and businesses, as well as through outdoor spaces like hillsides, city streets, and housing developments. Like the science of acupuncture, whose meridians map the flow of energy in the body, Feng Shui maps the physical environment with features that define energy flow in the natural world. Outdoor features such as hills, trees, rivers, roads, and buildings absorb and direct the energy flow in their area. Indoors, the windows, walls, furniture, and decor do the same.

Because energy flow is vital to—and synonymous with—life and health, Feng Shui seeks to identify or create places where energy flows freely and abundantly; these places then confer abundant energy to their inhabitants, who gain good luck, good health, harmonious relationships, and financial prosperity by being where the energy is. Conversely, an environment where energy flow is weak or obstructed may disrupt the inhabitants' energy balance to the extent that they may suffer ill health, domestic strife, or financial difficulties. Feng Shui is thus an art of nature and environment that links individual well-being with the health of one's surroundings.

A family might consult a Feng Shui practitioner if there are many fights in the house, for instance, or if one of its members is chronically ill. Shopkeepers commonly consult Feng Shui practitioners to improve business.

Dysfunctions in any aspect of health, harmony, or prosperity signal an imbalance in energy flow—often an imbalance in one or more of the Five

Elements. Feng Shui practice proposes specific cures for these imbalances, and may involve rearranging furniture, altering the landscape, or adding a strategic item like an eight-sided mirror or a red stripe to a difficult area. Like adding a new exit ramp to a highway, these alterations allow for new patterns in the "traffic" of energy flow. There are many styles of Feng Shui practice that dictate different varieties of ills and cures. Most of the suggestions in this book are derived from the work of the Black Hat sect of Feng Shui practice, as described by Sarah Rossbach and Lin Yun in their books on the subject.

One of the tools of Feng Shui is an eight-sided figure known as a Ba-Gua (see illustration). The Ba-Gua is a template—essentially a map—that connects specific sectors of a room or plot of land with certain areas of life—like health, wealth, etc.

In the practice of Feng Shui, the Ba-Gua is commonly superimposed on a room or home to determine which areas of the room correspond to which aspects of life. A western wall thus corresponds to the children in a household, while the southeast corner is affiliated with wealth. The walls and furnishings in these parts of a room can then be adjusted to improve the corresponding life areas. A western wall can be stimulated with specific Feng Shui "cures" (like a mirror or a plant) to encourage the conception of children, for instance, or to help existing children in the home with physical or emotional problems. While there are many different ways of using a Ba-Gua, this book presents a few simple strategies for tailoring a home to accord with Ba-Gua correspondences.

The chapters that follow show how the Five Element cycle contributes to the practice of acupuncture, dietary therapy, QiGong, and Feng Shui. Moving from the macro- to the microcosm, each chapter describes an element as it appears in the larger world, in nature, and in general cycles before focusing on the details of its presence in our bodies and in health. This structure was chosen so that by the time readers approach the most physical aspects of Chinese medicine, they will be able to see them as clear examples of the more general patterns. However, Chinese medicine itself makes no distinction between medicine and life: the human body is inseparable from the context in which it occurs. So for those who may be tempted to thumb through the "philosophical" sections of the book to get to the real medicine, remember that the philosophy *is* the medicine.

The specific exercises, examples, and recipes provided in each chapter are meant as suggestions only: there are infinite ways to rebalance your elements and the examples should serve as a springboard for your own creative experiments.

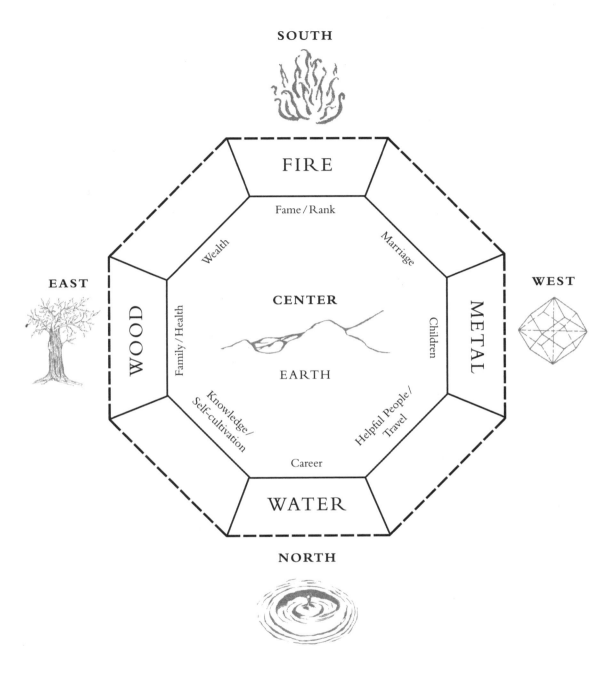

The Ba-Gua

Feng Shui maps and compasses traditionally place South at the top of the page—in contrast to the Western Style of locating North at the top.

Wood Becomes Water

Chinese Medicine in Everyday Life

CHAPTER I

ORIGIN

THE FIVE ELEMENT CYCLE THAT LIES AT THE HEART
of Chinese medicine is, at its core, the simplest of concepts—
a circle. The elements—Wood, Fire, Earth, Metal, and
Water—are stations of that circle.

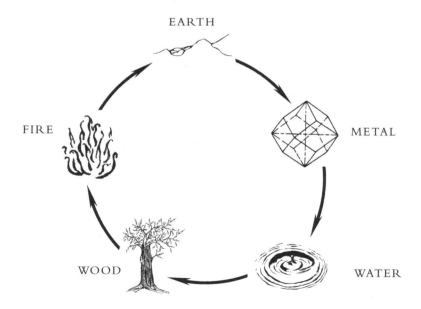

Like other circles since the beginning of time, the Five Element circle symbolizes the continuity of life. Without beginning or end, a circle is timeless, evoking the continuous renewals of night and day, the orbits of the planets, the phases of the moon, and death and rebirth. In cultures the world over, from ancient Europe to Asia, Africa, and the Americas, the circle has been used in ritual and in art to represent the continuous and cyclical nature of life.

Some of the first circles created by humans were drawn on cave walls during Paleolithic times (c. 35,000–9000 B.C.E.), where they are thought to denote fecundity, femininity, and creation. Round like the sun and moon, circles remind us of the totality of the cosmic creation. And, like the eggs that contain all of life, circles also evoke the microcosm.

Many ancient circles were used to mark time, describing its passage as an endlessly repeating cycle. Britain's great stone circles, for instance, like the one at Stonehenge, are monuments to the patterned movements of the sun and planets. As the planets make their yearly rounds in the sky, they become visible near certain stones in the circle at the same time every year. Elaborate rituals have been constructed around these patterns—like the dark chamber at Newgrange, Ireland, carved with intricate designs more than five thousand years ago. These designs were (and still are) visible only seventeen minutes a year, when the winter solstice sunlight enters the cave through a hole carved precisely for that purpose. The precision with which such events

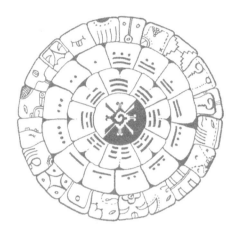

Mayan calendar

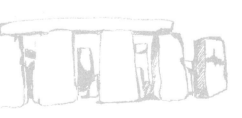

Stonehenge

were calculated indicates that these monuments were used as markers of ceremonial time.

Many ancient calendars were formulated as circles to convey a cyclical sense of time. The great Aztec sun calendar, for instance, is drawn as a circle. It integrates the cycles of the sun and moon and locates everything from crop rotations to astrological information within those cycles. The zodiacs of Europe, India, and China similarly unify in a circle the relationship of the sun, moon, and planets with human events. They testify to the regularity and circularity of both human and heavenly time.

Other circles describe internal or spiritual time rather than external time. These circles map the universe of inner experience, understanding that life is a journey or passage through which we all pass. The image of a labyrinth, carved and painted throughout ancient Europe, implies such a journey— often a descent into the underworld and a subsequent return to the world of the everyday. Such journeys impart wisdom to those who complete them.

Mandalas, likewise, map inner experience onto the physical domain of the circle. Tibetan sand mandalas have multilayered meanings, depicting the universe, the palace grounds of enlightened beings, a womb for the Buddha, the Five Elements, and a map for special meditative techniques, among other things.

Like a mandala, the Native American medicine wheel maps a variety of territories: the physical domain of the earth, the metaphysical domain of the spirits, and the inner domain of personal evolution.

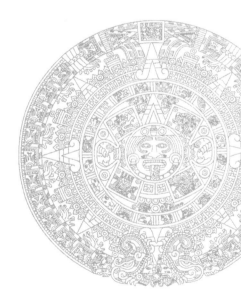

Aztec Calendar

Each direction (north, south, east, west) represents knowledge and understanding of a particular kind: Initiates go on internal "journeys" around the circle of the four directions, collecting the unique wisdom housed at each one. They become more and more whole with each step of the journey.

These cycles and circles are important because they identify both change and regularity as constant features of life. The passage of time, of journey, of growth, are changes laid like melody over the rhythmic repeat of our natural cycles; in combination they create a music that allows us to change and grow within ordered bounds. What shamans and healers have known since the beginning of time is that if we can learn to live in harmony with this natural music instead of fighting against it, we will strengthen our ties to the rest of creation. On a microcosmic level, this will lead to better health and longer life; on a macrocosmic level to harmonious relationships and a healthier planet.

Like other circles, the cycle of the Five Elements integrates human activity with the natural rhythms of the universe. The cycle has been used to map time like a calendar, space like a compass, the movements of the heavens, the divination of events on earth, medicine, psychology, music, and even the rise and fall of emperors. It is also used, like a medicine wheel, to map the internal journey of life and spiritual growth.

With so many ramifications, the Five Elements are not really elements in the classical sense (like the

Tibetan Mandala

four Greek elements), because they are not static materials. Instead, they are more like phases of a larger movement. In fact, the Chinese characters for the Five Elements are often translated as the five "movements," five "phases," or five "processes." Many practitioners prefer these translations, as they better connote the sense of movement that the cycle itself implies; however, the phrase Five Elements has become standard in the field, and will be used throughout this book in spite of its limitations.

The origins of the Five Element cycle lie in Taoism and the shamanic religions of ancient China. At times inseparably linked, both Taoist and shamanic practices emphasize Harmony with nature as a standard of living and as a foundation for ritual. The Five Element cycle most likely dates back to the second or third millennium B.C.E.—around the time of the ancient Egyptians. The oldest remaining records, however, come from the third and fourth centuries B.C.E., and are attributed to a man named Tsou Yen, whose work standardized thoughts that had apparently been widely used but chaotically interpreted up to that point. His writings established the Five Element cycle that is currently in use.

Tsou Yen's five phases—Wood, Fire, Earth, Metal, and Water—are drawn as a circle, and catalogue the stages of growth and decline inherent in all life processes. Wood represents birth and early growth, Fire pertains to the height of development, Earth describes transition and balance, Metal governs decline, and Water represents death and renewal. Living processes are considered to move through this cycle from Wood to Fire to Earth to Metal to Water, then back to Wood again, first growing, then declining, then renewing and growing again. The continuity of this cycle can be grasped most easily in relation to the cycle of the seasons, where Wood's early growth corresponds to spring, Fire's activity relates to summer, Metal's decline is akin to autumn, and Water's repose is like winter. Earth's transition is analogous to late summer, as well as the equinoxes and solstices, which are turning points in the seasons.

The cycle itself is considered to emerge from the universal whole known as the Tao. Usually translated as "the Way," the Tao is, however, unnameable and unfathomable. The

Tao Te Ching, the primary sourcebook of Taoism, tells us that "the Tao which can be spoken of is not the true Tao," because to speak of it betrays the inner knowing that characterizes it. The nature of the Tao is the subject of many works of philosophy, but for the purposes of this book the Tao can be understood, in part, as a kind of soup of universal essence. This soup creates itself continuously and exists at all moments, underlying and informing our manifest world. All things emerge from it and return to it, but the Tao itself has no particles, no planets, no life-forms. It is said to "give birth" to the Way, and through the Way to everything else in the universe; therefore the seeds of all objects, all creatures, all concepts, all time, and all space are melted together in the great universal Tao. It is the source and the wellspring of life as we know it.

The cycle of the Five Elements emerges from the Tao and expresses those aspects of it that are transitory and changeable. While the Tao itself neither transits nor changes, its manifestations on earth and in the heavens do both. The Five Element cycle is a testament to those changes, illustrating the patterns of change that are common to all life. More than a time clock, the Five Element cycle uses an elaborate system of correspondences to bring order and rhythm to a host of life experiences.

From its beginnings, the Five Element cycle connected various aspects of experience to its individual elements. Seasons, body organs, emotions, sounds, colors, directions, and climates were all

Collected together, the ethers of the universe constitute a unity; divided, they constitute Yin and Yang; quartered, they constitute the four seasons; [still further] sundered, they constitute the five elements. These elements represent movement.

—Tung Chung-Shu

distributed over the cycle of five. The Wood element, for instance, was said to correspond with the season of spring, the color green, the climactic force wind, the Liver and Gallbladder, the emotion anger, a sour taste, the east, and so on. The Fire element corresponded with the season of summer, the color red, etc. (See table below.)

These correspondences allow practitioners of Chinese medicine to diagnose and treat illness in a variety of ways, from emotional, physical, spatial, and dietary perspectives.

	WOOD	FIRE	EARTH	METAL	WATER
Season	Spring	Summer	Solstices and Equinoxes	Autumn	Winter
Direction	East	South	Center	West	North
Color	Green	Red	Yellow/Brown	White	Black/Blue
Climate	Wind	Heat	Dampness	Dryness	Cold
Sound	Shouting	Laughter	Singing	Weeping	Groaning
Emotion	Anger	Joy	Worry	Grief	Fear
Taste	Sour	Bitter	Sweet	Pungent	Salty
Yin Organ	Liver	Heart/ Heart Protector	Spleen	Lungs	Kidneys
Yang Organ	Gallbladder	Small Intestine/ Triple Heater	Stomach	Large Intestine	Bladder
Orifice	Eyes	Face	Lips	Nose	Ears

Although no one knows where the correspondences came from, they are the foundation upon which much of Chinese medicine is built. They are accepted as articles of faith, all the more so for having been borne out over thousands of years of practice. However, the correspondences themselves are only a part of the Five Element cycle. The other part involves theories about the way the elements interact with each other. When the correspondences are combined with the theories, the Five Element cycle becomes a system that can be applied to any situation. It demonstrates how body parts, people, creatures, and gods relate to one another.

The relationships between the elements are summarized below:

• *All things possess the Five Elements.* All objects, situations, and processes can be viewed in terms of the Five Elements.

• *Any phase of the Five Element cycle can be infinitely divided into its component parts.* For instance, in a twenty-four-hour day, morning is considered Wood, but morning itself can be divided into five more phases, such that dawn and waking are the most Wood-like aspects of morning, whereas getting up, dressing, and getting to work are more Fiery, and so on.

• *The Five Elements continuously create one another.* In the Five Element cycle, each element is said to create or be the "mother" of the one that follows it, and to be generated from (or be the "child" of) the one that precedes it. Wood, for instance, is created by Water, and is the creator of Fire. Fire creates Earth, Earth creates Metal, and Metal creates Water. This relationship is called the Creation cycle.

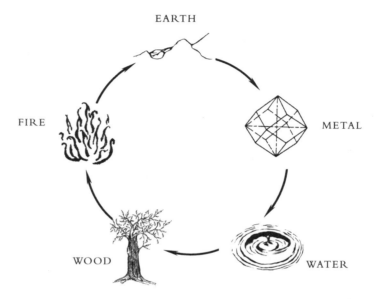

• *The Five Elements continuously consume and control one another.* This consuming and controlling acts as a balance to the Creation cycle, ensuring that no single element can grow excessively out of proportion to the others. On one hand, each element consumes the powers of its "mother" in order to exist. Water consumes the Metal that forms it and thereby keeps it in some degree of balance. However, the elements also exist along a Control cycle, which allows the elements to balance each other more actively. In the Control cycle, each element has the power to control and diminish another, just as it is controlled. Wood controls Earth, Earth controls Water, Water controls Fire, Fire controls Metal, and Metal controls Wood.

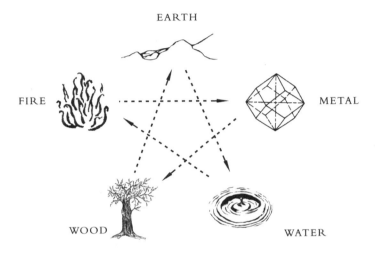

Together, the Creation and Control cycles specify the relationships that every element has with each of the others.

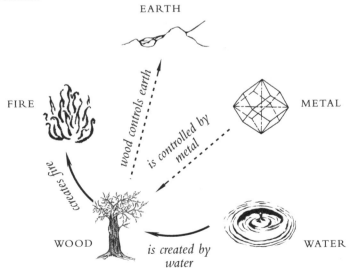

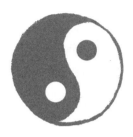

The Yin Yang symbol, also called the Taiji, illustrates the fluid interplay of Yin and Yang, which is governed by the same laws of creation applied to the Five Elements. One can see in the serpentine shapes the creation of Yin from Yang and Yang from Yin; how each contains within it the seed of the other (illustrated by the circles); how each consumes the other as it grows, and transforms into the other to create a continuous flow.

• *The Five Elements transform into one another, and each contains the seeds of all the others.* The lines between the elements are not hard and fast. What looks like Water according to one person's analysis may be classified as Metal by another's, or may mutate into Fire or Wood as conditions change. Because the cycle describes transformation, this mutability is an integral part of it.*

The above five "laws" of the Five Elements were originally construed to apply to another great cycle of Chinese thought—the polarity of Yin and Yang. Any exploration of Chinese medicine must include this duality, which telescopes the workings of the entire universe down to a single dynamic: the interplay of positive and negative. Also understood as masculine and feminine, or form and functional, aspects these generalities are not mere opposites, but complementary parts of any whole, like a top and bottom, a beginning and an end, the head and tail of a coin.

Every object, action, and quality is divisible into its Yin and Yang aspects, neither of which can be separated from the whole. Yang represents all that is expanding, moving, growing, bright, hot, masculine, active, while Yin refers to the forces of dark, quiet, condensation, introversion, and all that is passive, feminine, cool, and decaying.

* These five "laws" were originally applied to Yin and Yang in *The Web That Has No Weaver* by Ted Kaptchuk. I have taken the liberty of transposing them into the Five Element cycle.

YIN	YANG
shady side of a hill	sunny side of a hill
Earth	Heaven
cold	heat
moon	sun
passive	active
solid	hollow
feminine	masculine
receptive	projective
contracting	expanding
substance	essence
downward	upward
night	day
dark	bright

The polarity of Yin and Yang helped the Taoists to interpret the internal dynamic of all things. It added a dimension of subtlety to the ancient universe by presuming at least two sides to every truth. As all things possess Yin and Yang characteristics, Yin and Yang became a tool that could shed light on every relationship.

Although the Five Element cycle and Yin Yang doctrine developed separately, the two were often used together to describe natural phenomena. In some places they intertwined completely, and by the Han dynasty period (206 B.C.E.–221 C.E.), the emerging forms of Chinese medicine relied heavily on both systems. Viewed in combination with Yin and Yang, the Five Element cycle is like a further division of the primary duality; each element represents a particular proportion of Yin to Yang.

In this sense, Wood is considered the first element in the cycle. It represents early Yang—the beginning of a Yang phase. A child or an idea in the Wood phase of the Five Element cycle displays early Yang characteristics like birth and growth, expansion and youth. Fire follows Wood. It represents Absolute Yang—a stage in which movement and activity are as Yang as they can be; a planet or a story in the Fire phase is in a stage of climax and peak growth. Together, Wood and Fire make up the Yang half of the cycle.

Earth follows Fire. It signifies transition, and contains Yin and Yang in equal measure. Lives in an Earth phase are transforming from Yang into Yin.

Metal signifies early Yin. In the Metal phase, a flower or an ocean wave is no longer growing but has begun to consolidate and decay. Water is the phase of Absolute Yin. Creatures and events in the Water phase are absolutely at rest—no longer growing, no longer even decaying, but already dead or dormant and preparing for a new

beginning. Together, Metal and Water make up the Yin portion of the Five Element cycle.

The stages of ebb and flow described by the Five Element and Yin Yang cycles are aspects of all growth: They can be found in living things like humans and plants, in nonliving entities like civilizations and careers, and in creative processes like writing or building. The great wheel of life thus lends itself to many aspects of our experience, casting them as living systems with their own births and deaths, struggles and transitions.

The beginning of the Five Element cycle is the Wood phase, which finds qi in the process of condensing and taking on form. As Wood's voluminous energy bursts into being, the process of life begins.

You have noticed that everything an
Indian does is in a circle,
and that is because the Power of the
World always works in circles,
and everything tries to be round. . . .
The sky is round, and I have heard
that the earth is round like a
ball, and so are all the stars. The wind,
in its greatest power, whirls.
Birds make their nests in circles,
for theirs is the same religion as ours. . . .
Even the seasons form a great circle
in their changing, and always come
back again to where they were.
The life of a man is a circle from
childhood to childhood,
and so it is in everything where
Power moves.

—Black Elk,
Oglala Sioux

CHAPTER 2

WOOD

THE FIRST ELEMENT IN THE FIVE ELEMENT cycle, Wood, signifies creation—birth, life, and its subsequent evolution. A link between Heaven and Earth, the Wood element's creativity turns heavenly energy into earthly form. The trees that embody the Wood element are symbols around the world of creation and growth. Tammuz, the ancient Sumerian god of vegetation, was revered as the tree of life, while both life and knowledge were trees in Eden that represented the creative power of God. Christmas trees—and the pagan evergreens that preceded them—invoke the birth of light and the Lord during dark midwinter. In Japan, it is common to plant a cherry tree for every newborn child, while Israelis plant trees when people die, to ensure everlasting life in their name.

Both ancient Norse and Mayan peoples recognized a "world tree" as the central pillar around which the universe was organized. The Mayan Yaxché grew at the center of the world and, with its branches, held up the four corners of the sky. For Buddhists, the Bo tree (*ficus religiosa*) represents spiritual awakening, as it was under this tree that the Buddha attained enlightenment.

Ancient Celts honored trees as spiritual beings in their own right—each with its unique wisdom. Both the Celtic alphabet and calendar were based on tree names, so that time and all written knowledge were gifts of the tree spirits. In fact, the word for "trees" also meant "learning" in Celtic Irish. Particularly venerated was the oak—*duir*—which, as the king of the trees, marked the first letter of the Celtic alphabet (D), and the central month of the calendar, also known as Duir.

In the Five Element cycle, Wood symbolizes new beginnings—birth, growth, and development. It is the phase in which new lives take form and *become* something, like a sprout that draws wind, water, and light into a coherent stem. Defined in the Creation cycle as the child of Water, Wood emerges from the undivided whole and gives rise to the separation of individual forms. In the Control cycle, Wood is controlled by Metal, whose sharpness cuts through it and limits or directs its growth.

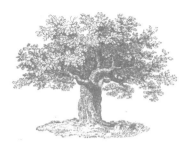

Duir (oak)

Beth (Birch)

The oak tree (above), called Duir in Celtic Irish, represents the central consonant of the Irish alphabet (D), and the central month of the traditional Druidic calendar. The Beth tree (Birch) is the first consonant of the alphabet and the first month of the calendar.

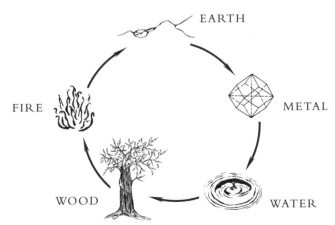

EARTH

FIRE

METAL

WOOD

WATER

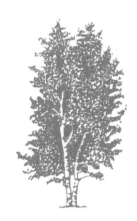

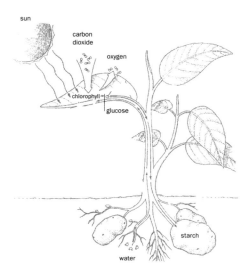

During photosynthesis, plants transform sunlight and water into starch—creating matter from energy.

In the natural world, trees link sky and ground with the many-fingered reach of their branches and roots. Holding fast at one end to the firmness of Earth, trees are yet able to bend and turn as conditions change around them; they reshape their trunks to grow toward the light, sway in the wind, and twist themselves around obstacles. This combination of firmness and flexibility is key to the trees' survival, and one of the hallmarks of the Wood phase. It allows for growth in relation to the surrounding environment, creating complex interdependent systems.

On a physical level, living things in the Wood phase transform energy (that was stored as potential energy during the Water phase) into matter. Photosynthesis in the plant kingdom is a perfect example of this metamorphosis. During photosynthesis, cells in green plants convert the energy stored in sunlight into carbohydrates, which form the solid leaves, stems, and roots of the plant. Because plants continuously transform energy into matter in this way, they exemplify the Wood phase, but anything growing relies on Wood energies, whether it's a muscle, a child, or a plan for a building.

In the cycle of the seasons, Wood corresponds to spring, when countless new forms are created from energies that rested, germinated, and hibernated through the cold winter. Seeds, bulbs, and buds explode into individual stems and fronds, while trees and plots that were bare yesterday are suddenly transformed by shoots and leaves. This growth—rapid and exponential—epitomizes Wood energy.

The explosion of life that springtime brings is found in animal as well as plant communities. A time of birth for many animal species (including most mammals and birds), spring is characterized by new lives. Animals that come out of hibernation begin new lives too as they emerge from a womb of sleep to restart the processes of survival. In spring, new forms and new beings are created every day.

Dawn heralds the Wood phase of a day—the morning that is born as the sun rises. Day takes its shape in the morning, as certain weather patterns adhere to it, and schedules, moods, and events come together to define it. Although conditions will certainly change as the day progresses, it is the very boundary of the dawn that defines the day and gives it form. It is Wood energy that governs this period of forming and defining, and Wood energy that we engage with as we plan each day and begin to play it out.

In the construction of a building, the Wood phase is in the planning stage—in choosing the site, drawing up the architectural plans, calculating and purchasing the materials. The building takes on its shape as the plans and materials are determined, just like a sprout beginning to take on the shape of the plant it will become. The building up of any new enterprise like a business or a baseball team is similarly a Wood phase.

The Wood phase of any creative idea—whether for furnishing a room, writing a story, planning a craft project, or making an investment—involves the brainstorming, planning, and research that define what is going to be done and how it will be achieved. From the moment an idea comes into consciousness until it is fully under way, Wood's creative energies predominate. Like other Wood-phase activities, the process of bringing ideas into reality is akin to birthing them; it brings their energy into form.

In this way, all creative activity is aligned with the Wood phase. Although the source of creative ideas lies in Water, the actions that bring them into being belong to Wood.

At first, any new idea or concept is formless—it emerges from the Water phase as a single idea. But the idea takes form as we embellish upon it, attaching images, plans, and specifications. This planning adds substance to the original spark. It is a process of growth and as such relies on Wood energies.

Similarly, the Wood phase corresponds to that portion of the menstrual cycle when the uterus prepares for the implantation of a fertilized egg. During days seven to fourteen (after the menstrual flow has stopped), the uterus builds up a thick inner lining that will support a fertilized egg, if there is one. Such building and preparation are signs of the growth that epitomizes Wood.

On a cosmological level, the Wood phase is analogous to the Big Bang—the birth of the universe—and the early rapid growth that gave rise to countless new life-forms within it. Physicists surmise that all the atoms—that is, all the *matter*—in the universe would have been created in the first few hours after the Big Bang. Such instantaneous creation marks a clear departure from the formless void that had existed previously; it characterizes the Wood phase in that the matter appeared out of nothingness. When form cohered out of formless energy, an entire universe was created: So explodes the power of Wood energy.

The supernatural forces of spring create wind in Heaven and wood upon the Earth. Within the body they create the liver and the tendons; they create the green color . . . and give the voice the ability to make a shouting sound . . . they create the eyes, the sour flavor, and the emotion anger.

—*The Yellow Emperor's Classic of Internal Medicine*

The climate associated with Wood is wind. Wind expresses Wood's energies in the grand drama of the cosmos; its powers of movement and direction play out the tension between firmness and flexibility on a super-human scale. In the language of weather, wind heralds change—the cosmic equivalent of flexibility. Its gusty blows carry seedlings and insects from place to place, changing the population of geographic areas over time. In fact, wind is an agent of change, bringing new ideas and rearranging old ones. Any new situation or idea that confronts us is a wind blowing in from the hinterlands; it challenges our Wood element to be flexible in growing to accommodate the new influence. The "winds of change" are the unpredictable events of life, the surprises that require us to alter our vision of ourselves and our plans.

When channeled through a particular source like a windmill or a mainsail, wind becomes a forceful tool that demonstrates Wood's creative and defining energies. Wind focused in this way creates power that can drive machinery or sail ships. But wind can also wreak havoc in the form of hurricanes and tornadoes. It can bring bitter cold windchill factors to an already freezing day, or exhausting Santa Ana winds to a parched climate. Wind's power unleashed brings chaos and destruction. In Chinese medicine, wind is also an agent of illness that carries colds and other germ diseases into a body whose defenses are weak. Wind penetrates the skin, most readily at the head, neck, and upper back; it can also cause tremors, or symptoms that migrate around the body like a wind whipping from place to place.

In addition to its external influence as climate, Wood also influences the inner universe of emotions and personality. In Chinese medicine, the emotions are inextricably tied to both the external environment and physical health: They can arise from climactic changes or physical diseases, and can also

Amidst the grassland

Sings a skylark

Free and disengaged from all things.

—Matsuo Basho

create diseases. On an emotional level, the Wood element expresses itself as vision and direction, channeling energies toward a particular focus. Like the trunk of a tree or the funnel of a tornado, Wood directs resources into a desired form. Whether what you want is a day to relax, a career as a lawyer, or a living room with a certain "feel" to it, directed Wood energy envisions a goal and propels the seed of vision forward into action. Positively expressed, Wood energy manifests as the courage of conviction, appropriate action, and the ability to hold one's ground.

Wood's strength is tested whenever our internal sense of direction is challenged, whether by argument, doubt, or circumstance. If we abandon our plans too easily, Wood lacks power within us, while if we cleave too stubbornly to mistaken or unwise plans, Wood is overly rigid. Ideally, however, Wood manages the tension between firmness and flexibility, allowing our rootedness to create a stable base from which we can bend.

Great leaders often have a lot of directed Wood energy—they envision on a large scale, bringing social, political, and cultural changes into form.

The Rev. Dr. Martin Luther King, Jr., for instance, had a vision (his "dream" on the mountaintop), which he strove to manifest in reality. His strength of vision and his determination are trademarks of a Wood personality; they powered his success and inspired the devotion of millions.

In its more problematic lights, Wood's emotion flares as anger and frustration. The emotion that corresponds to Wood in classical texts, anger can be thought of as strength without an appropriate channel; it sends us raging around like a directionless howling wind. We grow irritable and angry when we can't put our ideas into action, when we don't feel powerful, or when we're confronted with changes we don't want to make.

Often anger arises when our sense of self has been compromised—when we feel we have been overlooked, disregarded, or deliberately thwarted. These situations offend our Wood element because it is Wood that supports our individuality and ego; if we feel we have not been treated with proper respect, Wood rears up and declares itself—through shouting, stomping, or aggressive behavior.

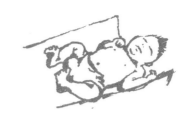

Anger may also flare when situations move beyond our control, failing to work out according to our dictates. Whether it's our plans for dinner, our jobs, or our habits, circumstances that meet with failure trigger Wood's emotions. Wood often finds us groaning like a stiff branch when the winds of change come howling through, holding on to anger rather than giving in to change.

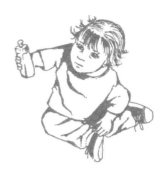

WOOD IN THE HUMAN LIFE CYCLE

In the human life cycle, the Wood phase spans birth through childhood. Before birth, fetuses are attached and entirely dependent. They are interior, suspended, and completely merged with the mother. At birth, however, babies separate from the mother and become individuals with distinct physical form and singular governance over breath, digestion, and excretion. This transition from interior dependence to external independence is a miraculous change, and one that perfectly illustrates the movement from the all-is-one union state of Water to the individual-being stage of Wood.

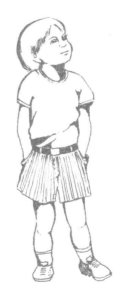

The rapid growth of childhood embodies Wood's expansive evolution.

Babies and children convert energy into matter daily, adding inches, pounds, and shape to their growing bodies. Although people grow continuously throughout their lives, they do so particularly quickly during childhood, embodying Wood's rapid and material growth. Children grow dramatically in other ways as well during the Wood phase, developing emotional, intellectual, and spiritual capacities and values. Our unique personalities—complexes as well as capabilities—grow in response to stimuli from the world around us.

Emotional growth can be compared to the way plants bend toward the light and roots shape themselves around rocks in the soil. Such adaptations evolve through profound interweaving, as plants and animals slowly shape themselves to accord with their surroundings. These organisms do not merge with their surroundings, succumb to them, or overpower them; rather, they grow *with* those surroundings, *because* of them, into the unique selves they are destined to become. Emotional development is much the same, in that children grow personalities that reflect the unique circumstances of their upbringing. Wood's role in this development is to maintain integrity while supervising change, balancing—as always—the tension between firmness and flexibility.

The spirit of the Wood element is aspiration*—the ability to envision one's future in the world with hope and excitement. Aspiration anticipates Wood's growth, encouraging and, at times, even creating it. It calls us forward toward our highest and best selves, like all attributes of spirit. Spirit is a Yang and striving influence that inspires perfection and everything that is most godlike in us. When Wood's spirit of aspiration is lacking or dysfunctional, depression ensues. Those who suffer from it have no sense of hope or forward motion, and feel themselves to be losing impetus instead of growing.

The Wood phase of soul development refers to the process of becoming conscious as an individual: developing a sense of self based on inner knowing and individual truths rather than on externally imposed standards. As distinct from spirit, the soul does not strive toward the future; instead, it digs deep inside to find out who we are at this moment. Whereas the spirit holds the image of our highest selves, the soul mirrors our most confused and human selves. It teaches us to become

---

* The discussions of soul and spirit in this work are separate from the classical discussions of the five "souls" that correspond to the Five Elements. The information presented here on the soul and spirit of each element is drawn from my own work, and is not a part of classical Chinese medicine.

whole through the sweat and minutiae of hard work and human suffering, effecting growth as we recognize our limitations and labor honestly with them.

During the soul's process of becoming more whole, called "individuation," we become more fully ourselves, peeling away the layers of what society or our parents or our own striving spirits push us to become. Though it begins in childhood, individuation continues on through early adulthood, and for some people throughout their entire lives. It involves discovering inner truth and becoming responsible toward it, shaping one's economic, social, and personal life to reflect it. In the hard work of making us true to our deepest internal selves, however, the soul often causes profound pain; we find ourselves doing things the "hard" way, though it flouts logic, advice, domestic harmony, and our own sense of honor.

Because the Wood phase is more about individuation than about connecting or partnering, it often takes form as the more difficult aspects of a relationship: conflict and resistance. Individuals in a Wood phase struggle to define themselves, to maintain their boundaries, and to ensure that outside forces don't overwhelm them. They want to get their needs met, and to feel like active agents in the world. Therefore they resist incursions and demands from others, often deliberately challenging other people as a way of testing their own strength. This struggle for definition frequently becomes a struggle for power, because we presume that the strength of our

In the spring sea

Waves undulating
and undulating

All day long.

—Yosa Buson

parents or partners interferes with our own. We mistakenly look for external causes for our feelings of powerlessness and subsequent dissatisfaction, not recognizing that it comes from within.

Although the parent or partner is rarely an actual obstacle to growth, our Wood phases often bring resentment of them. We believe we are not growing because "they" are not giving us the space. An adolescent resenting his parents' involvement in his life typifies this scenario, but it happens as frequently in adult relationships, when friends or partners compete with each other for attention, power, or independence.

The truest way through such a period is to recognize the internal need to express oneself more fully, to pay attention to inner truth and knowing. When Wood rears its head as frustration and resentment, it is a call to pay attention to one's inner power, intuition, and goals. At its best, this phase allows people to grow as individuals so that they bring more complete selves to all of their relationships.

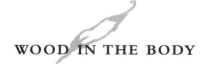

WOOD IN THE BODY

In the body, the Wood element expresses itself through the organs of the Liver (which is considered a Yin organ) and the Gallbladder (a Yang organ). Together, these organs govern all qualities associated with Wood in human life, like growth, creativity, newness, individuation, etc. They also have specific functions within the body, which form the basis of much of Chinese medicine's diagnosis and treatment strategy.

The Liver rules smooth flow. The expression of Wood's flexibility, smooth flow is the physical correlate of "taking things in stride." It ensures that our emotions and energies adapt to the many changes we face on cellular and experiential levels. This aspect of the Liver keeps emotions, qi, and blood running smoothly in the body; when it becomes dysfunctional, symptoms like moodiness, anger, and pain can result.

The Liver stores Blood. Blood in Chinese medicine is the physical expression of a sense of self. It nourishes and moistens our self-esteem, providing a rich understanding of who we are, much like the process of individuation. Through its management of Blood, the Liver nourishes and moistens muscles and tissues, regulates menstruation, and provides a foundation for the Heart and Mind.

When an imbalanced Liver is unable to properly store and nourish Blood, the body may develop scanty menstrual periods, a pale and dry complexion, numbness, or poor self-esteem.

The Liver controls the sinews and manifests in the nails. Sinews, including tendons, ligaments, and skeletal muscles, create the body's shape. As healthy sinews result in toned and flexible musculature, this aspect of the Liver manifests Wood's affiliation with form and strength. In addition, the overall health of the Liver is reflected in the smoothness, strength, shape, and coloring of finger- and toenails.

Imbalances in these functions of the Liver can create muscle spasms or tremors, muscle weakness, or yellowed, cracked, and malformed nails.

The Liver opens into the eyes. The Liver's association with the eyes exemplifies Wood's qualities of vision and direction. In this capacity, the Liver governs visual acuity, maintains moist and clear eyes and eyelids, promotes inner vision and direction, and rules clairvoyance.

When ill or dysfunctional, this aspect of the Liver can cause vision problems, eye diseases, or a lack of inner vision.

The Liver absorbs what can't be digested. Just as the Wood element builds up anger at situations that can't be controlled, the Liver stores ingested substances that can't be directed. It regulates the levels of fats and sugars in the blood, converting them into storage molecules when they over-burden the bloodstream, and it collects residues of alcohol, coffee, tea, tobacco, and other drugs (prescription, over-the-counter, and recreational types), as well as pesticides and other chemicals in our foods.*

When the Liver is overburdened, its role in digestion is compromised, resulting in blood-pressure or blood-sugar imbalances, constipation or slug-gish stools, addictions, and anger.

The Liver controls immune response. The body's allergic and immune responses enact, on a cellular level, the drama of distinguishing self from other. Just as the Wood element defines and protects our personal boundaries, this aspect of the Liver defines and protects our chemical boundaries, identifying and expelling foreign invaders.[†] When the Liver is unable to perform this function, immune and autoimmune diseases can arise, like allergies, arthritis, multiple sclerosis, etc.

The Gallbladder rules decisions. The Gallbladder rules that aspect of Wood energy that makes choices. It elevates to conscious awareness the processes that lead to evolutionary and adap-tive changes—like whether we should "grow" this way or that way, go to the movies or stay home and read.

Dysfunctions of the Gallbladder can therefore result in indecision.

The Gallbladder makes and stores bile. The only Yang organ that stores anything (storage is a receptive and

---

* This is not one of the functions of the Liver in classical Chinese medicine, but has been adopted by many modern practitioners in recognition of the substantial evidence supporting this interpretation found in modern scientific and alternative health therapies. Since the development of Chinese medical theory predates the use of refined and synthetic foods, the buildup and storage of such substances would not have been an issue in Classical times.

† Like the Liver's absorption functions, immune response is a quality that is not a part of Liver function in classical Chinese medicine. However, it is included here because it has been found to correspond with the general health of the Liver.

Yin function), the Gallbladder stores bile and assists the Liver in the digestion of fats. When the Gallbladder is compromised, fats can accumulate in the bloodstream or tissues.

On the surface of the body, the Wood element manifests in the meridians of the Liver and the Gallbladder. These meridians distribute Wood's energy from head to toe, and contain the points that allow acupuncturists to regulate the functions of the Liver and Gallbladder organs. The meridians can also register imbalances *before* they get to the organs. These organs can be treated to prevent or slow the development of organ disease.

The Liver meridian begins on the big toe and runs along the inner aspect of the leg. It runs through the genitals and up the trunk to end on the chest below the nipple.

The Gallbladder meridian begins at the outer edge of the eye and traverses the sides of the head and trunk to end on the outside of the fourth toe.

WOOD OUT OF BALANCE

Imbalances in the organs or any of their functions can occur for a number of different reasons. External factors such as extreme weather or invading germs can throw an element off balance, but so can emotions, imbalanced food intake, or insufficient rest. Alternatively, an element may be dragged or pushed

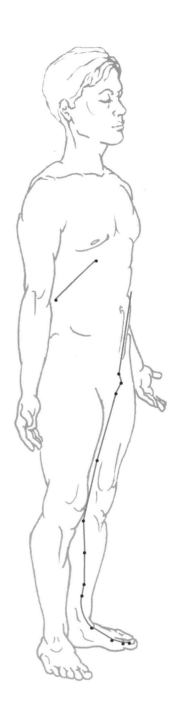

Liver Meridian

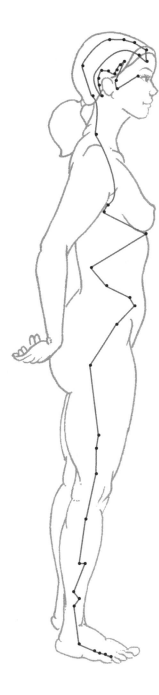

Gallbladder Meridian

out of balance by another element in the cycle.

When an element loses its balance, its functions may become more pronounced, or less so. In Chinese medicine, such imbalances are referred to as either *excesses* or *deficiencies*. This means that the qi within the element is out of balance and teetering between extremes. Corrective measures—like those described later in this chapter—regulate the balance of qi and harmonize the relationship among all the elements. When an element is deficient we *tonify, strengthen,* or *support* it, while treatments for excess *disperse, reduce,* or *sedate.*

Wood in Deficiency

When an element is deficient, its functions will be weak. When Wood is deficient, it may be deficient in one or more of the functions described above—in its Blood-storing capacity, its control of the eyes, etc. Common symptoms of Wood deficiency include:

- ★ blurred or weak vision
- ★ deficient immune response
- ★ passive behavior
- ★ scanty menstruation
- ★ dry skin
- ★ tremors or numbness
- ★ low self-esteem
- ★ cold hands and feet

- ★ incomplete individuation
- ★ inability to make decisions

Other signs may include pale complexion, dizziness, restlessness, dry or discolored nails, low blood pressure, a lack of creative interest, a lack of adaptability, dry eyes, severe depression, or muscle weakness as occurs in multiple sclerosis and neuromuscular diseases. On a creative level, deficient Wood manifests as an inability to move from Water into Wood—one can't come up with ideas, or comes up with ideas only, which never get translated into action. A person who is a "pipe dreamer" is a classic deficient Wood type—always talking about "someday . . ." but never taking action.

When a Wood deficiency is the primary imbalance, the other elements may also be pushed or dragged out of balance. Over time, for instance, Wood may lose the power to nourish its child in the Creation cycle, which becomes weak. Or Wood may become unable to control its subordinate element in the Control cycle, which then rears up into excess. The following diagram illustrates the most likely patterns of imbalance that result from a primary Wood deficiency.

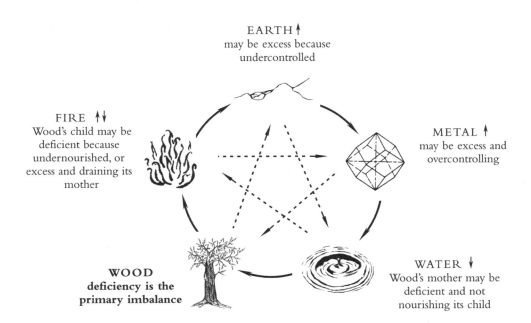

EARTH ↑
may be excess because
undercontrolled

FIRE ↑↓
Wood's child may be
deficient because
undernourished, or
excess and draining its
mother

METAL ↑
may be excess and
overcontrolling

WOOD
deficiency is the
primary imbalance

WATER ↓
Wood's mother may be
deficient and not
nourishing its child

An Example of Wood Deficiency

Donna M.'s daughter brought Donna to acupuncture for treatment of her Parkinson's disease. At seventy-one years of age, Donna suffered from tremors in her hands, and was starting to exhibit spasticity in her movements. Her face and lips were very pale, her hands and feet cold, and she often suffered from dizziness. In addition, Donna's behavior in the treatment room was very distinctive. She had a hard time talking about herself, and would always steer her dialogue toward praise of her daughter, whom she felt worked very hard, yet was taking this time to bring Donna to my office. Donna asked several times if she was seated in the wrong chair, and repeatedly offered that chair to her daughter and to me, though we were both comfortably seated.

Donna suffered from a weak Wood element, which manifested with deficient Liver and deficient Blood signs. Tremors are a classic sign of wind—Wood's climate—and although they can be caused by a number of factors, in this case it was the Liver's inability to properly store and nourish the Blood. Improperly nourished Blood also caused other signs of Blood deficiency in Donna—pale face and lips, dizziness, and cold limbs. Her behavior demonstrated a marked Wood deficiency as well—a passive and self-abnegating attitude that rendered her unable to talk about herself, and unable to feel that she deserved her daughter's time or even a chair to sit in. Although Donna's lack of a sense of herself was extreme, many people suffer Wood deficiencies in similar ways.

Treatment for Donna would focus on strengthening her

Wood element—particularly in its Blood-storage capacity. In addition, Metal would be dispersed to prevent it from overcontrolling Wood.

Wood in Excess

When Wood (or any element) is in excess, its functions may become exaggerated, while excess energy and fluids can build up and cause pain, heat, phlegm, inflammation, etc. These excesses may overflow into Wood's child in the Creation cycle, causing excess in that element as well. At the same time, excess Wood is very likely to overcontrol its subordinate in the Control cycle, leading to a deficiency in that element.

Common signs of Wood excess are:

* moodiness/irritability/depression

* high blood pressure

* anger

* PMS

* menstrual cramps

* rigidity or spasticity

* allergies/hyperimmune response

* inflammation

* gas, constipation, diarrhea, nausea, hiccups, or belching

* pounding headache

According to the inflationary model, the universe had a brief period of extraordinarily rapid expansion, or 'inflation,' during which its diameter increased by a factor of at least 10^{25} times larger (and perhaps much larger still) than had been previously thought. In the course of this stupendous growth spurt all the matter and energy in the universe could have been created from virtually nothing.

—Alan Guth and
Paul Steinhardt,
The New Physics

Other symptoms include pain, itching, itchy or red eyes, lack of energy, shortness of breath, violent behavior, stuffy head or chest, tendinitis, difficulties in bending and stretching, Bell's palsy, and stiffness. Creatively, a Wood excess will show up as someone who plans extensively but has trouble actually getting down to work.

When a Wood excess is the primary imbalance, the other elements may displace as follows:

EARTH ↓
may be deficient because
overcontrolled

METAL ↓
may be deficient and
undercontrolling

FIRE ↑↓
Wood's child may be
deficient because of
energy stoppage, or excess
because overflowed into

WATER ↓
may be deficient because
drained by child

WOOD
**excess is the
primary imbalance**

Mercedes K. is a good example of Wood excess. She came to acupuncture for treatment of chronic migraine headaches. Several times a week Mercedes was plagued by pounding headaches on the right side of her head, which made her dizzy and nauseous, and which disrupted her vision. The pain was so severe that she was often bedridden for hours. When asked to pinpoint the site of her pain, Mercedes located Gallbladder meridian points on the side of her head and above her eye. She also suffered from premenstrual moodiness and ovarian pain during ovulation.

Upon examination, Mercedes's Gallbladder meridian was extremely tight and sore to the touch in several places. This is an excess in a Wood meridian. The nausea was caused by overactive Wood invading Earth, while the dizziness and pounding were signs of Liver Blood rising up instead of flowing smoothly. Ovarian pain and premenstrual moodiness are also signs of Liver not maintaining a properly smooth flow of qi, Blood, or emotions.

Treatments for Mercedes would begin with dispersal of her Wood excess. In conjunction with this, however, one would tonify her Earth element so that it could better withstand Wood's overcontrolling.

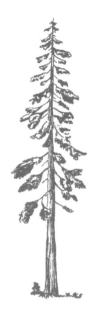

Redwood tree

Cases of combined excess and deficiency can occur when the flow of energy is blocked between an element and its child in the Creation cycle. In this case, excess builds up in the mother element because it can't get through to the child, which then becomes deficient. In a more complicated scenario, a pronounced excess or deficiency over a long period of time can mutate into its opposite—prolonged rage (excess) can collapse into severe depression (deficiency), or numbness and dizziness (deficiency) can transform into a pounding headache (excess).

WOOD AND ACUPUNCTURE

In acupuncture, imbalances in the Wood element may be treated through the Liver and Gallbladder meridians, in combination with other strategies.

These meridians, like each of the twelve main meridians, have points on the limbs that correspond with each of the Five Elements. With special needling techniques, the Five Element points can be tonified or dispersed (or treated neutrally) to affect the Wood element's dynamic within the cycle.

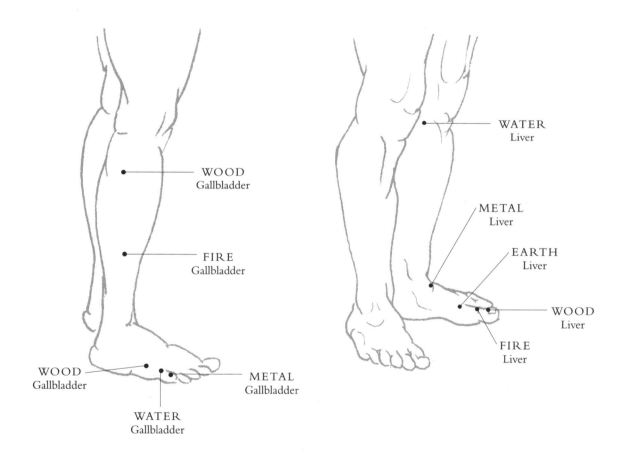

*Detail of Five Element points on the
Gallbladder and Liver meridians*

The **Wood** points on the Wood meridians have a particularly strong effect on the Wood element. They can be used to tonify deficiencies or to disperse excess.

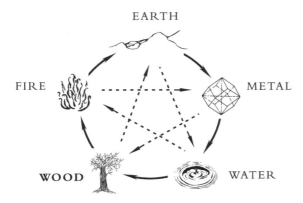

The **Fire** points on Wood meridians are commonly used to subdue excess Wood that has raged out of control, overflowing into excess Fire.

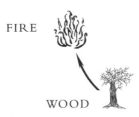

The **Earth** points on the Wood meridians are used to affect the relationship between Earth and Wood. They are commonly used for syndromes of Wood invading or overcontrolling Earth.

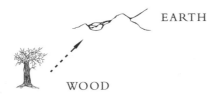

Be like a tree in pursuit of your cause. Stand firm, grip hard, thrust upward, bend to the winds of heaven, and learn tranquility.

—Dedication to Richard St. Barbe Baker, Father of the Trees

The **Metal** points on the Wood meridians affect the relationship between Metal and Wood. If Wood is excess, showing the signs and symptoms described above, tonifying these points will help Metal control Wood.

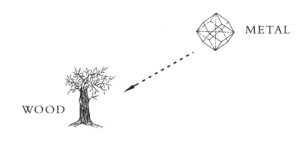

The **Water** points on Wood meridians influence the dynamic between Wood and its mother, and are therefore especially useful for tonifying deficient Wood. They can also be used, however, when excess Wood drains its mother, and when excess Water overflows into Wood.

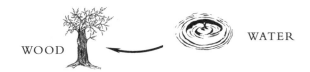

Common treatments for Wood deficiency involve Wood and Water, its mother, as well as Wood's controlling element, Metal. Water points on the Wood and Water meridians will tonify Wood through its mother, while Metal points on Wood and Metal meridians stop Metal's over-control of Wood.

Donna M., described earlier, was treated with such points to strengthen her Wood element. Over time, her spasticity disappeared and her tremor grew less pronounced, while her complexion grew rosier. Donna also began to show signs of a developing sense of herself. She began to talk about her own emotions during her visits, and to ask directly for things that she needed—a glass of water, a blanket, etc. One day she even scolded her daughter for interrupting her!

A treatment for Wood excess would include Metal, Wood's controlling element, and Fire, Wood's child. Metal points help Metal control Wood, while Fire points help drain Wood through its child.

During Mercedes's course of treatment, her headaches stopped almost completely. Every couple of months she might get a headache or feel as if she was about to get one, but these would go away if she took aspirin or a nap. No longer driven by her anger, Mercedes's entire manner changed; her voice grew softer, she stopped scowling, and her outfits began to look put together as opposed to ill-matched and startling. She started a new company and began to plan her financial future. As her Wood element grew back into balance, Mercedes was able to integrate more comfortably into her world, envisioning her goals and even putting them effectively into action.

WOOD AND FOOD

The Wood element manifests in the foods we eat with its distinctive flavor, shape, and color. The plant kingdom, in general, is aligned with Wood because plants embody Wood's growth, Wood's greenery, and Wood's transformation of energy into matter. All vegetables, and green ones in particular, therefore, carry an ethos of Wood energy along with whatever other characteristics they may have.

The foods eaten during Wood's season, spring, also affect the health of the Wood element, as does the quality of the foods we eat, since the Liver absorbs the toxins (from chemicals) and excess metabolites (from sugar and fat) that are not immediately used by the body.

Wood's flavor: sour

Wood's flavor is sour. Sour cools the body, consolidates energy, and astringes fluid. (Astringence draws and tightens tissues. It is what happens in your mouth when you eat a lemon.) Note, however, that consolidation shrinks things down, and astringency draws them away: These functions are opposite from the growing and expanding qualities one normally associates with Wood, and are consonant with the Metal element instead. This is because flavors enter organs according to the Control cycle. Metal controls Wood, so Metal actions like consolidation penetrate Wood, affecting its energies by opposing them. Flavor energetics work largely through the Control cycle in this way, and it is because of this controlling function that overeating a particular flavor will quickly weaken its associated element.

Sour foods penetrate the Liver and Gallbladder, stimulating them and affecting their energy flow. Small amounts of sour foods can thus be added to a diet when the Liver and Gallbladder are in excess or deficient, though large amounts will certainly weaken them. Examples of sour foods are lemons, sour plums, yogurt, hawthorne berries, limes, pickles, and sauerkraut. Other foods are predominantly sour, but secondarily associated with another flavor as well: Vinegar is sour and bitter, for instance, and leeks are sour and pungent, while aduki beans, apples, blackberries, cheese, grapes, mangoes, olives, sourdough breads, and tomatoes are all considered sour and sweet. Sour herbs include rose hips, sumac, and purslane.

Wood's vegetables: stalks*

Foods that grow upward on strong stems and stalks embody Wood's image of growth, and therefore have a connection to the Wood element. Foods in this category include asparagus, wheat, corn, and celery. These

---

* Information about Five Element correspondences with food shapes and growth patterns is inspired by the work of Jeffrey Yuen.

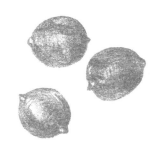

foods have a strong Yang and rising energy, and they are good for symptoms of Wood deficiency.

Wood's fruits: berries

Berries have strong astringent and diuretic properties—like Metal—and are therefore appropriate for controlling Wood excesses. Berries include strawberries, raspberries, cranberries, and blueberries.

Wood's color: green

All green vegetables have a special affinity for the Wood element. They can be used to tonify deficiency and control excess, although strongly deficient people should eat them well cooked and in combination with more warming foods.

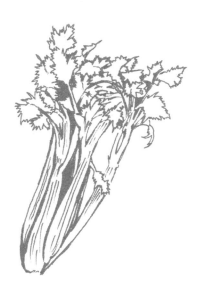

Tonifying Wood Deficiency

To tonify Wood deficiency, eat Wood's vegetables, along with sweet (Earth) and salty (Water) foods, as described in those chapters. Since Wood is the first Yang element in the cycle, a Wood deficiency is also often associated with Yang deficiency, resulting in cold and pale limbs and a lack of energy. Therefore foods with a warming thermal nature, as described in the Fire chapter, will also be helpful. Because Metal controls Wood, Metal foods should be avoided.

Roasting foods also helps to tonify Wood deficiency by warming and expanding body energy. Roasted vegetables and meats are traditionally associated with fall and winter feasts because their warmth helps to offset the chill of the colder seasons.

Lemons are associated with the Wood element through their sour flavor. The upright stalks and green color of celery make it a wood-element food as well.

WOOD-DEFICIENCY RECIPE
Beef with Asparagus, Watercress, and Cracked Green Peppercorns

5 tsp. fresh lemon juice

9 tsp. olive oil

$\frac{1}{4}$ tsp. sea salt

$1\frac{1}{2}$ lbs. beef tenderloin cut into
    5 equal pieces and flattened to
    about a quarter inch

3 tbsp. dried green peppercorns, coarsely
    ground with a mortar and pestle

10 asparagus stalks, lightly steamed and
    chopped into 1-inch slices

2 cups watercress leaves

1. Mix the lemon juice, olive oil, and salt in a small bowl and set aside.

2. Heat a large skillet over high heat until very hot.

3. Meanwhile, coat each piece of beef on both sides with the peppercorns. Place in the pan and sauté until medium rare, about 30 seconds on each side.

4. Remove and plate the meat, and turn the heat to low. Add 2 tsp. of the olive oil/lemon juice dressing and toss the asparagus and watercress in the skillet briefly, until they wilt. Drizzle them with the remaining olive oil dressing and serve alongside the beef. Serves 5.

Wood Excess: A Diet for Spring

During spring, the Liver and Gallbladder are naturally active and have a tendency toward excess. People at this time of year are often somewhat congested internally from winter's slow pace and heavy diet: They're especially likely to manifest with Liver-excess symptoms, such as allergies, irritability, restlessness, anger, indecision, and constipation.

A diet for spring, or anytime Wood excesses need to be reduced, should include a fair amount of sour foods as well as plenty of green vegetables. Since the Liver collects so many impurities during digestion, sour's purifying function is crucial to cleaning and clearing its excesses. The sour flavor draws impurities out of the Liver (astringing them) and acts as a solvent upon them, breaking them up so they can be eliminated.

Bitter and pungent foods, as described in the Fire and Metal chapters, can also be included. (If Wood excess has created a lot of heat, however—manifesting with Fiery symptoms like infections, headaches, or outbursts of anger—the more warming pungents should be avoided.) Spring meals should emphasize Wood's lighter Yang and rising qualities and should be the smallest and the lightest of the year. Salty and heavy foods, like sweet and fatty ones, are best left uneaten.

A diet that supports the Wood element, whether excess or deficient, should above all be *clean*—the more fats, sugars, alcohol, coffee, chemicals, and dairy products we eat, the more we exacerbate any existing Wood imbalances. While these "problem foods" tend to be the ones we turn to in times of stress and depression, they give their temporary comfort at the expense of long-term health, and do more damage than most people realize. As difficult as it may seem at first, removing these items from the diet will likely heal a large part of whatever ails you.

As a prelude to cleaning up the diet, many people like to undertake a fast or a modified fast to accelerate Liver cleansing. (A modified fast may be eating only one kind of grain, or only vegetables, or only clear soups for a few days.) In early spring, or whenever the Liver is overly congested, a fast combined with the olive oil/lemon juice cleanser described in the sidebar is a great way to facilitate Wood's recovery.

WOOD-EXCESS RECIPE
Liver Cleanse
To be taken once or twice a year:

Fast or eat lightly for several days and ingest a mixture of two tablespoons of extra virgin olive oil and the juice of half a lemon or lime (or one tablespoon of apple cider vinegar) first thing in the morning. This process draws toxins out of the Liver so they can be eliminated, and after three to six days of it the whole body feels renewed.

This is also a good remedy for depression, though it should not be taken for more than a week.

WOOD AND QIGONG

Wood's strength is a product of its firmness tempered by flexibility—a result of the Liver maintaining smooth flow.

The physical exercises of QiGong evoke Liver's flow and wind's motion, and control body Energy, which is the QiGong treasure most closely aligned with the Wood element. In the East, where movement is used to prevent the stagnation that is a precursor to disease, movement has long been considered essential to health. QiGong tradition draws on two classic books of exercises—*The Muscle/Tendon Changing Classic* and *The Brain/Marrow Washing Classic*. The latter is more appropriate to the Water element, but the exercises of *The Muscle/Tendon Changing Classic* direct themselves clearly toward the sinews and tendons governed by the Wood element.

The movements of QiGong exercises are particularly well suited to Wood, as they flow smoothly, continuously, and regularly. (This applies as well to other contemplative exercises like Yoga and Tai Chi.) These exercises stretch the muscles and connective tissue, bringing moisture, blood, and vital nutrients to every nook and cranny of the body. Many QiGong exercises begin with a posture known as the horse stance. As an exercise in and of itself, the horse stance helps us to create free flow within the body. It establishes a perfect balance between firmness and flexibility. When used as a starting posture for other exercises, the horse stance roots the body stably and strongly—like a tree—thus creating a firm foundation for subsequent movements.

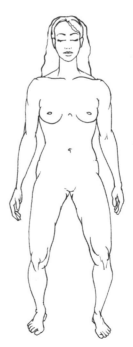

Horse Stance

HORSE STANCE

Place feet flat on the floor, shoulder-width apart, with toes turned out at a forty-five-degree angle. Relax the knees and bend them very slightly, just enough to prevent them from locking. Pull in the buttocks, tipping the pelvis slightly. Drop the shoulders, straighten the spine, and pull the abdomen in slightly. Elbows should be slightly bent, and the hands should hang loosely without any tension in the fingers. The head should be drawn up—as if suspended by a string from its top to the ceiling. In this position the chin will naturally tuck in a tiny bit, which helps keep the upper vertebrae straight. Eyes and mouth should be relaxed and gently closed. Keep the tongue lightly pressed against the roof of the mouth and the jaw relaxed.

Once in position, try to let your body's center of gravity drop to the ground and below. Feel your feet rooting in the ground like a tree. Try to place as much of your feet in contact with the ground as possible. Try to feel the texture and the temperature of the floor. Feel the earth pushing up against your feet and supporting you. Distribute your body weight along the thighs and center it equally on both feet. You may want to rock gently from side to side, and from back to front, in order to feel the distribution of body weight. Then try once again to center and balance it.

While rooting and centering the lower body, don't let the upper body collapse. Remember that it is being pulled toward the heavens as firmly as the feet are pulled into the earth. Visualize each vertebra lifting and separating; feel how firmly the spine supports the entire trunk, which expands and relaxes with each breath.

As an individual exercise, practice standing relaxed in the horse stance for ten minutes at a time.*

* Adapted from Yang Jwing-Ming, *The Root of Chinese Chi Kung*.

While people with Wood excesses may find themselves drawn to more active exercises like aerobics, sports, or running, maximum benefit is achieved by combining such a program with the stretching exercises of QiGong or Yoga, as they provide a good workout and cleanse and tone the body's organs.

WOOD AND FENG SHUI

Outdoors, the Wood element is present in trees, grasses, and all growing things. The health and abundance of the Wood element at any site reflects the nature of the qi there, such that strong healthy trees reflect good qi at the site, while scraggly growth or weak plants reflect the opposite.

In addition, trees have some specific associations in Feng Shui practice, and can be used for a variety of purposes in that context.

Because of their strength, trees can be used to screen a dwelling from evil qi that might be stalking it. For instance, a house with a river or road running straight toward it is normally considered vulnerable to the onrush of energy from such a river. But a screen of trees or bamboo stalks will shield the house from that unwanted "arrow" of energy. Similarly, trees can be used to screen out other "evil" influences at a site, like harsh rock formations or a sharp dropoff.

A screen of trees or a mountain is recommended at the north or northeast section of a plot to screen out the evil influences that traditionally come from that quarter. Trees themselves can attract bad qi if they are planted near the front gate, or they can obstruct wealth from entering the house if they are too near the front door.

Mountains or buildings with a tall, squared-off top are aligned with the Wood element. The World Trade Center towers are prime examples of Wood structures, as are most tall office buildings. (Pointed towers—like the Empire State Building—belong to the Fire element.) Architecturally, columns also evoke the Wood element.

Indoors, green is the color associated with Wood in the Five Element cycle. Like the green-growing plants that characterize the Wood phase, green represents expansion, growth, and activity. Green can occur in the wardrobe—

If the Wood element needs tonification in your life, try adding or emphasizing green in your wardrobe, your home, and your work space. Wear it, or place some green things in your field of vision. Softer, lighter greens are better for anger and other Wood excesses; brighter greens will help stabilize you if you feel whipped around or otherwise deficient. If you need to make a major change, replace metal or plastic furniture and implements with wooden ones. In addition, you can paint a picture with lots of green in it, buy green socks, shop for vegetables, borrow a book with color photographs of trees from the library. Be creative—green can be found in lots of places! Because plants represent a balanced Wood element, it's a good idea to spend some time with them. Bring home a new houseplant, explore green grass and leafy trees, go to a botanical garden, or just gaze at a potted plant. Also see the Water chapter for tips on tonifying Wood through its mother.

If you have a Wood excess, try to remove greens from your life for a while. Hide or remove whatever green things you can, and make a point of not wearing green until you feel more balanced. While it is unnecessary to get rid of wooden furniture or other household items, there are other things you can do. Make or buy white or metallic pillows for that green couch (Metal controls Wood), buy brass or copper candlesticks or other decorative items, repaint the walls if their white has dulled or faded. Because trees represent balanced Wood energy, houseplants or a walk in the woods are as helpful for Wood excess as they are for deficiency. (Also see the Metal chapter for more tips on tonifying Metal.)

as garments or as accessories—in upholstery, paint, artwork, crockery, floor coverings, and any number of incidental items like stationery, writing utensils, candles, bottles, etc.

Green is a good color for a desk or a study, as it helps to focus energy and concentration. It is especially good for children, whose mental energy is easily scattered.

Another way that Wood appears in the home is in the furnishings and decorations. The shapes, function, and material composition of furnishings all contribute to the health of Five Element balance. *Wood shapes* are tall and columnar, growing like a tree. Standing lamps, candlesticks, columns, and moldings are all examples of wood shapes, as are houseplants and trees. *Wood colors* are green and green-blue. *Wood materials* include anything made of wood—like desks, shelves, picture frames, doors, window frames, and floorboards.

The area of the Ba-Gua that corresponds to the Wood element is the east. This area also corresponds to family and to health. If there is discord in a family, try hanging a crystal or a red ribbon on an eastern wall, place a large, healthy plant there, or a mirror, or a favorite work of art. While these cures can be added to the eastern wall of any room, they would be especially helpful in a family room, for example, or in a doctor's office, where healing would be especially affected by this area of the Ba-Gua.

The southeast corresponds to wealth, which can be stimulated by adding a healthy green plant or red ribbon to a southeast wall or corner.

The three months of spring denote genesis and release. Heaven and earth are renewed in every respect; the ten thousand things blossom forth. [He who desires to order his life in accordance with this season] goes to bed at night and rises early. He moves through the house with powerful strides. His hair hangs freely

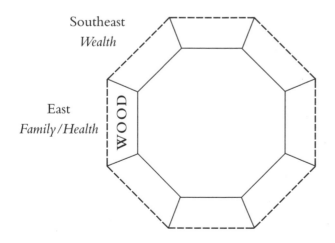

Southeast
Wealth

East
Family / Health

WOOD

down the back of his neck; he
grants his body the serenity
of true relaxation. In this
manner he is able to
cultivate his mind. To create, not
kill; to give, not take
away; to reward, but not
punish; these are [the actions]
in accord with the influences
that [embrace men]
in the spring, signaling the
correct way to bring
into existence [all things].
He who acts contrary
to these [influences] shall
harm his liver.

—*The Yellow Emperor's Classic of*
Internal Medicine

A healthy Wood element creates a person who is sure of himself and can speak up for his needs, but who also knows when to relax his urge for control and go with the flow. With stable and appropriate moods, the healthy Wood person reacts with steadiness when problems arise. He decides what needs to be done, plans accordingly, and puts his plans into action.

The lessons of the Wood element are evident in the trees that so eloquently express its character. Like the individuals we strive to be, each tree has its own form and identity, which becomes more distinctive with the weathering of every storm and more itself with each passing year. The rings that record a tree's history invoke the strength, steadfastness, and power to endure that are the hallmarks of a mature Wood element. With its roots in the ground and branches reaching toward the sky, a tree joins Heaven and Earth in a gesture of aspiration and uncompromising grace.

As we move through the powerfully defining energy of the Wood phase, we acquire a strength and a momentum that were lacking up to this point. Firmly rooted, we are able to reach higher and farther than before; our focus shifts as we begin to explore the world around us. Engaging with others, we enter the flaming territory of the Fire phase.

CHAPTER 3

FIRE

FIRE IS A SYMBOL OF DIVINITY, OF TRANSFORMATION, and of passion. In many world mythologies (Greek, Polynesian, Native American), fire is a power of the gods stolen by or for humankind. The only element that people can produce, fire reminds us that we, too, are creators; it symbolizes that which is godlike in us.

Long associated with divinity, fire often signals the presence of God. Lightning accompanies visions and prophesies in myths and stories, while the Old Testament's burning bush speaks in the voice of God. Around the world, the fires of church candles, temple fires of the ancient Greeks, and Kiva-fires of Native Americans manifest the presence of the gods in the houses devoted to their worship.

Also in this regard, fire is a potent symbol of purification. Christians have used it to burn away sins (and heretics), and the ancient Assyrians spoke incantations into ritual fires to disempower the acts of sorcerers. As symbolized by the phoenix (whose name means "red"—the color of fire), fire portends the resurrection that occurs after purification.

But fire is also a symbol of destruction: the fires of hell are punishments for sinners, while Pele, the Hawaiian goddess of the volcano, burns to death those who displease her. Old Europe's fire-breathing dragons personified evil, burning cities and stealing virgins. Evoking its destructive powers, we often use fire words to describe things that drive us to the absolute limits of endurance—unimaginable pains like holocausts, hells, and crucibles.

In world literature, fire is nearly synonymous with the burning of desires, be they physical, emotional, intellectual, or spiritual. These images of fire tell of feelings so powerful that they are utterly consuming.

In the Five Element cycle, the Fire phase describes a stage of peak power. Whereas the Wood element describes birth and a process of becoming, Fire celebrates that which has become. In the Creation cycle of the Five Elements, Fire is the child of Wood: It consumes the fuel of Wood to engage fully in the activity at hand. In the Control cycle, Fire is controlled by Water, whose stillness dampens Fire's consuming ardor. On a physical level, the Fire phase converts all available energy into kinetic energy, manifesting the full potential of a given system.

Fire, then, is about peaking—reaching a maximal stage of activity. Anything at its most active point—a motor at full throttle, an orgasm, a runner on her way to the finish line—is in a Fire phase. The English language has many expressions that describe the Fire phase, as in the "peak

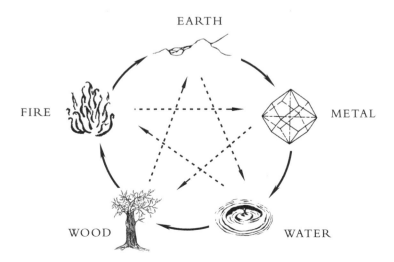

EARTH

FIRE

METAL

WOOD

WATER

of one's power," "full throttle," "full tilt," and "full steam ahead." As these expressions connote, Fire is a phase of doing the utmost, of maximal energy output, and of projects and cycles reaching their apogee.

What's important to recognize about the Fire phase is that it has a direct connection to the phases that precede it in the cycle; a Fire must burn *something* up, so it is only as powerful as the potential that was stored in the Water phase and activated in the Wood phase. Peak manifestation occurs when all the potential is realized—when all stored reserves are in play, on full burn. Rocket scientists work actively with Fire energies as they plan to launch a rocket. The amount of fuel required depends upon a precise calculation of the speed and intensity at which it will burn: Too intense a burn and the rocket may explode or overshoot its destination, too slow a burn and it will undershoot. At the edge of the Fire phase, there is little room for error.

In the cycle of the seasons, Fire corresponds to summer. Summer flowers explode from buds, embodying Fire energy in their brightness, their expansion, and their delirious proliferation.

Insects dart and buzz continually until the air itself seems to be in motion, while butterflies duck and rise like flames. Through it all, light and heat bear down with an intensity that sears the senses.

There is nothing subtle or hidden about summertime—everything's out there on display. Every potential flower and leaf comes fully into being; nestlings and fledglings leave the quiet shelters of their homes for the wider world. Thick furs and feathers give way to softer, lighter undercoats, and even the seldom-seen bodies of humans are exposed, as they pare down to the barest essentials.

In the cycle of a twenty-four-hour day, the full daylight hours are the most Fiery time. This is when the majority of people work their hardest, channeling energy into concentration, activity, and production. Whether in an office, a classroom, a home, at physical work or play, adults and children engage their creative and active energies most fully during this time.

In constructing a building, the Fire phase is the time when the building goes up. Beam is laid upon strut and cement is laid upon beam, and the work proceeds at a steady and active pace using the materials and plans accorded during the Wood phase. At this stage, the building is a work-in-progress, and will continue under its own momentum (as long as the resources don't get jammed or used up). In the Fire phase, things are in almost perpetual motion.

In any creative endeavor, Fire predominates when a project is in full swing—when a painting, a story, or a financial investment has become its own thing. At this stage, projects appear to take on lives of their own as they accrue according to an internal logic rather than the plans that began them. In this stage people may be "fired up" with excitement— devoting intense concentration to their work, staying awake for long periods, even losing track of time. Such behavior is emblematic of the Fire element in the intensity of its "heat," and in the powerful attraction it holds over the senses.

In the natural world, Fire as an element has distinct characteristics: It spreads, often covering millions of acres if left unchecked; it consumes, swallowing the vitality of all living things in its path; and it destroys. But fire can also be an agent of renewal. If allowed to burn naturally, forest fires remove old layers of plant life and allow more timid native plants to begin their growth.

In the Five Element cycle, Fire is associated with the animal kingdom, which consumes and digests the Wood of the plant kingdom. (The carbohydrates that plants form from sunlight make up fifty to eighty percent of most human diets.) Within the animal

Gargantuan clouds during dog days

Take the shape of a demon

Then change into the Buddha.

—Kobayashi Issa

kingdom, humans are the most Fiery of the Fiery: We consume the most fuel—animal, vegetable, and mineral (in the form of fossil fuels); engage in the most activity—building structures over the whole planet, and moving around over vast expanses of territory; we have even appropriated fire as a tool, directing it in the form of heat, electricity, combustion engines, and industrial power to the service of our Fiery tasks.

Note, however, that as beings of Fire we also exhibit in the extreme Fire's destructiveness. Like wildfire out of control, our restless consumption of resources and products devours everything in our path.

On a cosmological level, the Fire phase corresponds to the expansion of the universe that occurred just after the Big Bang. It is thought that the initial production of helium and other elements—the creation of universal matter that epitomizes the Wood phase—would have stopped after a few hours. After that, the universe is believed to have simply expanded for a million years or so, before the stabilization and forming of galaxies began.* This expansion is typical of a Fire phase, as it involved an almost random inflation of particles, which caused the universe to spread like wildfire.

In the menstrual cycle, the Fire phase corresponds to ovulation—beginning around day fourteen of the cycle. Rising levels of estrogen peak at this time, initiating the production of luteinizing hormone, which triggers ovulation. This is the Fiery peak of a woman's fertility cycle and the time when she is most likely to conceive; for many women, ovulation also marks the peak of sexual desire.

In any endeavor that actually involves fire or heat as a part of its process (like cooking, pottery, soldering or forging metal, etc.) the Fire phase is the portion of it that involves fire. When cooking or baking, for instance, Fire is active when the pan goes into the oven or onto the stove and the dish begins to cook. The potter's fiery kiln embodies Fire, too, as it cooks and transforms clay into a solid vessel.

Fire employed in this way is an agent of transformation; it alters the

* Trinh Xuan Thuan, *The Birth of the Universe: The Big Bang and After.*

inner structure of materials and changes them into something else. Baking *changes* the quality of the ingredients it cooks, turning batter into cake, and eggs into soufflé. Similarly, a forge transforms iron into a malleable state, so it can be shaped, reshaped, hammered, and reborn. In the Fire phase, forms transcend their original natures and may become something else entirely, or may temporarily merge and blend with each other.

The ancient study of alchemy relies on the transformational properties of Fire as its primary tool. In alchemical traditions, the earth's primary matter, combined with a catalyst, cooks in an oven and transforms (over time) into gold (whether actual or metaphorical). The magical Fire that achieves the structural shift is not just a material fire: The process does not work unless the alchemist who performs it is pure, devout, and devoted to his task. He must apply the "fires" of his own being in order to achieve transformation.

Though physical alchemy was and is practiced, its vocabulary and imagery are important symbols of emotional and spiritual transformation as well. Many mystical practices, as well as Jungian psychology, use the symbolism of alchemy to describe internal transformations. It's a metaphor for qualitative change, allowing us to transform pain into growth, envy into joy, or fear into love. Ancient Taoist traditions also describe a sexual alchemy— a process of transforming sexual energy into life-prolonging energy.

All that is living burns. This is the fundamental fact of nature. And Moses saw it with his two eyes, directly. That glimpse of the real world—of the world as it is known to God.

—William Bryant Logan,
*Dirt: The Ecstatic Skin
of the Earth*

In this sense, the Fire phase is a forge that changes the essential nature of whatever goes into it. Projects transform into realities, ingredients into meals; emotional fires like grief and love transform into wholeness. Creating new states of matter and transcendent moments of awareness, the actual and metaphorical fires of the Fire phase burn and transform reality.

The supernatural forces of summer create heat in the Heavens and fire on Earth; they create the heart and the pulse within the body . . . the red color, the tongue, and the ability to express laughter . . . they create the bitter flavor, and the emotions of happiness and joy.

—The Yellow Emperor's Classic of Internal Medicine

The sun contains and creates Fire energy in our solar system

The Fire element expresses itself climatically as heat. Like Fire, heat is Yang by nature, moving upward and outward. It speeds things up and promotes both activity and transformation. In our world we encounter heat from many different sources: sunlight, heavy clothes or blankets, warm drinks, exercise, fire, heated rooms and cars, furnaces, lights, and stoves.

Heat is essential to life and growth. It promotes movement and catalyzes the chemical exchanges that define the process of life. Heat warms the planet from without and helps break down ingested foods within, rendering nutrients absorbable by the body. It takes only a ray of sunlight on a cold day to realize how important heat is to life.

Too much heat, however, will destroy life. Living things wither in extreme heat, becoming dehydrated, feverish, and eventually moribund. In Chinese medicine, heat has very specific effects on the body. It speeds up the pulse and heart rate, can give rise to flushing, reddening, or inflammation, and to hot areas of the skin (like hives or infected areas). Because heat rises, it tends to manifest in the upper body—the trunk and head. Headaches, fevers, a flushed face, rapid heartbeat, and a stuffy feeling in the chest are all signs of heat. Infections and burns, both "heat" diseases in Chinese medicine, can spread rapidly out of control, consuming everything they touch.

On a more abstract level, heat is generated in the larger environment by excess. Overcrowding, noise pollution, environmental toxins, and information overload are some examples of this type of "hot" influence. One way of under-standing this idea is to imagine a room at a perfect temperature. Then imagine the room slowly filling with people; as it gets crowded, the temperature rises. There's just not enough room for air and people to circulate properly, so their energy builds up as heat.

Fire on an emotional level corresponds to joy and excitement. In its proper measure, joy warms, activates, and enlivens the body. Joy brings light to the eyes and an animated energy to movement; it opens the heart, and inspires people to connect in warm ways with friends, colleagues, and lovers. Joy also spreads—smiles and laughter are contagious, and people who are happy enjoy spreading happiness to others.

Chinese medicine also recognizes a state of too much joy, however—or too much excitement. It occurs when excitement becomes an all-consuming occupation that interferes with other activities. Conditions referred to in our culture as anxiety, hyperactivity, and hysteria are examples of this kind of excess fire. Inappropriate laughter, speech, movement, or behavior are all signs of excess heat and excitement, as are rapid heartbeat, flushed face, and red eyes. Manic disorders and the effects of caffeine and other stimulants also epitomize excess fire.

Jonathan M. is a good example of someone with chronic excess joy. Friendly and outgoing, Jonathan speaks in a nonstop streak, jumping from one topic to another often without apparent logical links. Interspersed in his patter are many jokes (often bad puns or sexual innuendo), which he laughs at merrily before continuing on to the next sentence. He even laughs at sad points in his monologues, discussing his symptoms or painful romantic entanglements—not recognizing that laughter at these moments is inappropriate. Jonathan doesn't really like to sleep, because it interferes with his late-night club-hopping "fun." Even on the acupuncture table, where most people sleep or trance out, Jonathan keeps talking. Pursuing acupuncture for treatment of his panic attacks, Jonathan suffers heart palpitations, anxiety, and difficulty breathing—all Fire symptoms.

Joy and excitement are physical as well as emotional experiences. They cause energy to rise in the body—like fire—away from the legs and solar plexus into the chest and head. This rising energy removes us from our bodies and pushes us into our heads; fantasy and anxiety are symptoms of this overbalancing—they are "head trips" that consume volumes of ungrounded energy.

Appropriate joy is a different matter. Like a good, deep belly laugh or keenly appreciated fun, healthy joy feels good in the whole body—it doesn't give rise to hysteria and a false speeding up, but actually slows things down. Great vacations and particularly fulfilling days feel long and rich in hindsight—appropriate joy expands time by opening the heart to greater levels of experience.

FIRE IN THE HUMAN LIFE CYCLE

In the human life cycle, the Fire phase is symbolized by adolescence and early adulthood, when the human being isn't just growing, but transforming—expanding in depth, intellectual capacity, and in relationship to the world. Adolescents are transformed by the Fire phase as hormones trigger sexual development and desires. Physically, the development of body hair, breasts, and beards symbolizes the spreading and expanding nature of fire.

Adolescents transform socially as well, forming intense friendships and/or romantic relationships that are often more powerful than their family ties. Beginning to reach out into the world, adolescents may find jobs outside the home, pursue outside activities that interest them, and develop personal expertise in physical, intellectual, or social endeavors. At this stage, young adults deepen their emotional, intellectual, and experiential selves, transforming into profound and independent creatures.

Desire—one of the hallmarks of the Fire phase—comes sharply into focus at this time of life. Unlike children, whose needs are usually quickly forgotten, teenagers are absolutely driven by their desires: for independence, for someone who understands them, for peace and social justice, for love, for knowledge, for sex, for freedom, and for the meaning of life. These restless desires cause teenagers endless amounts of pain, but also prompt them to reach out into the world in an effort to find satisfaction.

Desire typifies Fire in that it seeks to consume, to transform, and to merge. Sexual energy is a form of desire that perfectly epitomizes the Fire phase—it not only pushes us to reach out, it also hungers to merge with another being. This merging with another—and the physical intercourse that accompanies it—is a fire within Fire.

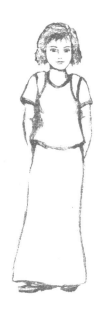

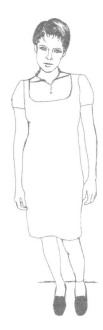

Adolescent transforming to a young adult

A catalyst for emotional growth, Fire is vitally important to the spirit, for it leads toward transcendence—Fire's spiritual attribute. Just as Wood's spiritual attribute, aspiration, points us toward our highest and best selves, transcendence calls us toward our highest levels of experience and understanding. When we transcend our mundane selves, we join with the forces of creation, seeing the world as the gods see it, understanding in a brief flash what they understand always.

There is a moment when an object on fire transcends its physicality and becomes air, smoke, and ash; the spirit on fire similarly transcends its human limitations and becomes divine. Worshipers transfixed in prayer, shamans in ecstatic dance, and lovers in sexual union all experience moments of complete transcendence, when they release their private forms and unite for an instant with the Creation that made them.

Although such moments of union between spirit and the divine are brief, they create a lasting echo of faith, which assures us we can have such experiences again. Faith is the knowledge that union exists, and it is an attribute of the Fire element for its promise of transcendence.

On a soul level, Fire is the element of connection. The Fire of the soul prompts us to find communion with others, to appreciate our same experience, to find that we are not, after all, so different. In connection we find a joining; it is the instant of meeting someone's eye, of sharing the same joke, of uniting for a common goal. Whereas transcendence unites us with God, connection unites us with other earthly beings. We might feel connected to our pets, to the sad-eyed gorillas we see at the zoo, to our ancestors. Connection reminds us that we are all one soul.

Real connection happens, however, only after real individuation, for it is only when we understand who we are that we can understand what we share with another. True self-awareness results in real love: romantic love, familial love, and compassionate love for the other beings sharing this lived experience.

On a relationship level, Fire mediates between outreach and letting people in. In one sense, all relationships take place in a Fire context, because it is Fire's desire to connect that is the impetus behind the relationship in the first place. Fire is the desire for union that propels us to seek out others. In friendship or in romance, this desire for union is usually the first stage; it invites a seeking outside of the self for a connection with somebody else.

Fire and the Heart

The organ mainly associated with Fire—the Heart—has strong affiliations with love and relationship in myth and language all over the world. Indeed, it is the Heart's power of emotion and connection that permits one person to relate to another at all. The Heart strives for union and finds joy in the experience. The more unity, the more love; the more joy the Heart finds, the more it radiates these delights to others. Like a glowing hearthfire, the Heart spreads warmth and intimacy to all who come within reach.

The Western world has a long tradition of connecting the heart with love, although the currently dominant scientific model has shifted the seat of emotions to the brain. In Chinese medicine, however, the Heart remains a center of emotion and of spirit. In fact, the Heart is said to "house" the spirit,

so that the emotions and passions that penetrate it actually run both deeper and higher; they allow relationships that transcend the earthly plane and connect one to the divine. Fire's consuming passions—for other people, favorite foods, particular activities—create such strong feelings in us because they connect us to the divine through the aegis of the spirit.

The Heart gives love, but it also receives love by allowing others to enter its most private territories, which is the greatest act of faith a human can perform. In our Heart centers, others have the power, not only to heal us with their love, but also to destroy us if they should deny or abuse that love. In this way, the Heart is our most vulnerable organ: It must be open in order to receive what it needs, yet its openness contains the seeds of despair. It is a paradox that terrifies all who honestly consider it, and which prevents many people from accepting the love they crave.

Fire and the Small Intestine

The Small Intestine, a Yang Fire organ, separates truth from untruth. It sorts

Fire moves:
elk and bison run
before the wind.
Fire jumps canyons
and grizzly
bears' den sites and
flies over shaky-
legged oxbows . . .
Flame builds
to massive walls; it
gathers whole
forests with
double-jointed
arms, laying down
life as ash.

—Gretel Ehrlich,
Islands, the Universe,
Home

beliefs and precepts of self-awareness, discerning which hold true in one's "heart of hearts" and which should be discarded. The source of our "gut" feelings, the Small Intestine screens our thoughts for us, determining whether "I'm sorry" or "I love you" is true before we say it.

Fire Energy and the Heart Protector/Triple Heater

Because the Heart remains, of necessity, vulnerable to sorrow, the body has constructed strong defenses for it. A second pair of organs—the Heart Protector and the Triple Heater—accompany the Heart and Small Intestine in the Fire element. (This is unusual; Fire is the only element in the cycle that governs two organ pairs.)

The Heart Protector surrounds the Heart and protects it from unexpected hurt and violation. Filtering the influences that beg access to the Heart on a continuous basis, the Heart Protector evaluates the potential for harm of a given person, remark, or action and allows only acceptable risks to pass along to the Heart.

An important part of this protective function is monitoring the emotional trustworthiness of people around us. The Heart Protector allows us to open ourselves up to those who demonstrate themselves to be responsible toward us, but prods us to withdraw and wait when there are confusions or violations of trust.

In established relationships, the Heart Protector

governs our willingness to be open, our presence and honesty in the relationship, and our response to being hurt. When a friend, partner, or sibling says something cruel or thoughtless, the Heart Protector closes us down. Outwardly we may withdraw, get angry, or grow teary as a private door swings shut inside, preventing further remarks or deeds from penetrating to the Heart. It is the Heart Protector, too, that releases us from our self-imposed isolation when the environment is safe again. Apology and forgiveness are themselves Heart activities, but it is the Heart Protector that allows us to speak the apology, or to let someone else's explanation penetrate to our own heart to engender forgiveness.

The Heart Protector also acts as a filter for our psychic input, keeping our Hearts from being overwhelmed by the thousands of signals that other people broadcast about themselves. Like a sensitive satellite dish, the Heart Protector collects information about the people we encounter—a new business associate, for instance—and determines whether they are hostile or friendly,

strong or weak, stable or volatile, dangerous or warm. Though the frequencies are rarely discernible to the naked eye or ear, the Heart Protector reads them clearly and opens or restricts access to the Heart accordingly.

The Triple Heater gauges everything from the actual temperature in an environment to the safety of the building we stand in. It is the Triple Heater, for instance that intuitively gauges the "vibe" of a room, deciding whether it feels comfortable, safe, or awkward.* The Triple Heater also governs those psychic abilities that are more external than personal—the ability to predict stock market activity, political changes, airplane crashes, etc.

FIRE IN THE BODY

In the body, the Fire element expresses itself through the Yin organs of the Heart and Heart Protector, and through the Yang organs of the Small Intestine and Triple Heater. These organs are responsible for the outreach,

* This explanation of the role of the Triple Heater derives from the work of Lonny S. Jarrett, in particular from his article "Chinese Medicine and the Betrayal of Intimacy" in *The American Journal of Acupuncture,* Vol. 23, No. 1, 1995.

connection, and exuberant energy that characterize the Fire element. The Heart has a special place among the organs, however, and is considered to be the supreme ruler of all of them, compared in ancient texts to an emperor seated on his throne.

The organs of Fire also have the following physical functions :

The Heart governs the Blood. Whereas the Liver's Blood management regulates self-awareness, the Heart's Blood nourishes self-love. It shines the light of the Heart's love and joy onto our perceptions of ourselves. The Heart makes Blood and circulates its warming fires through the body's network of vessels and capillaries.

When this function of the Heart is disturbed, there may be fatigue, insomnia, anxiety, dizziness, lack of love, or a disturbed spirit.

The Heart controls the pulses. A primary diagnostic tool in Chinese medicine, the pulses are controlled by the Heart that circulates blood through the vessels. While specific pulse positions indicate conditions of the organs, the strength, regularity, and smoothness of the pulse overall reveal the quality of Fire's energy—the constancy of the Heart. Dysfunctions in this aspect of the Heart may manifest with weak, erratic, or irregularly timed pulses.

The Heart houses the spirit. The spirit lives in the Heart, which thus maintains the emotional connection between humanity and the divine. It is the source of the fires that transform our lives. If the Heart is sufficiently or continually imbalanced, the spirit cannot adequately root within it, and becomes disturbed.

Signs of disturbed spirit include insomnia, poor eye contact, inappropriate speech and laughter, mental illness. (See QiGong section p. 80 for more about the spirit.)

The Heart manifests in the face and opens into the tongue. Faces reveal the emotions of our Hearts: An open expression signals trust and openness, while a tight face indicates the opposite. In addition, the brightness, elasticity, overall moistness, and coloring of the facial complexion reflect the quality of Heart blood and its circulation.

The color, shape, and moistness

of the tongue are governed by the Heart, and the speech facilitated by the tongue indicates the state of our Heart's spirit. In this way speech patterns, stuttering, and hesitations reveal imbalances of the Heart.

The Small Intestine separates the pure from the impure. The Small Intestine inherits partially digested food and drink from the Stomach and separates out the purer food and fluid essences. It then releases purer essences to the Spleen, and impure products to the Bladder and Large Intestine for elimination. The psychological correlate of this process is the separation of true (or "pure") thoughts and beliefs from untrue ones.

Dysfunctions of the Small Intestine can create irritable bowel disorders and an inability to trust one's own judgment.

The Heart Protector wraps and protects the Heart. Like a prime minister who protects the emperor, the Heart Protector protects the Heart from overstimulation and emotional shock. It also receives and screens psychic impulses.

When the Heart Protector is overburdened, it can cause anxiety, palpitations, and erratic commitments to others, with a tendency to overtrust and undertrust at alternate times.

The Triple Heater divides the body into three sections. The Upper Heater includes everything from the diaphragm upward, including the Lungs, Heart, ribs, throat, head, and brain.

The Middle Heater comprises everything between the diaphragm and the navel, and the organs of the Spleen, Pancreas, Stomach, and Gallbladder.

The Lower Heater is everything below the navel, including the organs of the Liver (considered a part of the lower burner because of its meridian affiliation with the sexual organs), the Large and Small Intestines, Kidneys, Bladder, uterus, and sexual organs.

The Triple Heater distributes Source qi. The Triple Heater distributes a form of primal qi energy known as Source qi, which is produced by the Kidneys and has a catalyzing effect on all the other qi transformations in the body.

The Triple Heater controls the Water passages. The Triple Heater mediates between Fire and Water, helping to

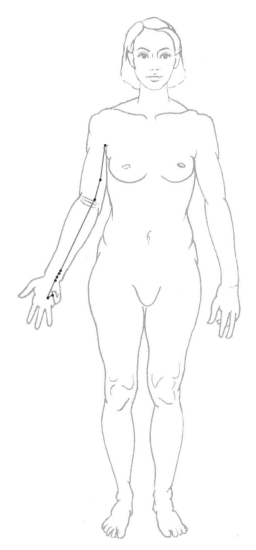

The Heart Meridian

distribute and disperse water and fluids in the body.

The Triple Heater governs the interrelationship among organs. The Triple Heater connects all the organs together and distributes energy among them.*

On the surface of the body, the Fire element manifests along the meridians of the Heart, the Small Intestine, the Heart Protector, and the Triple Heater.

The Heart meridian begins in the chest and runs along the inner aspect of the arm to the palm of the hand and the pinky finger.

The Small Intestine meridian begins on the pinky and runs up the underside of the arm, along the top of the shoulder blade, and up the side of the neck before ending in front of the ear.

The Heart Protector meridian begins on the chest and travels through the armpit and along the inner aspect of the arm and palm, ending at the tip of the middle finger.

The Triple Heater meridian starts at the tip of the ring finger and travels up the back of the hand and arm to the top of the shoulder. It then goes up the side of the neck and around the ear to end at the outer tip of the eyebrow.

* Some suggest that the Triple Heater corresponds to connective tissue in Western anatomy and physiology—a provocative notion, as the connective tissue's prevalence and function in the body accord with the Triple Heater's in many ways: Connective tissue, or fascia, wraps every organ, every vessel, and every muscle, tendon, and nerve in the body. Literally connecting every part of the body to every other part, connective tissue has also been found to conduct bioelectricity (like qi).

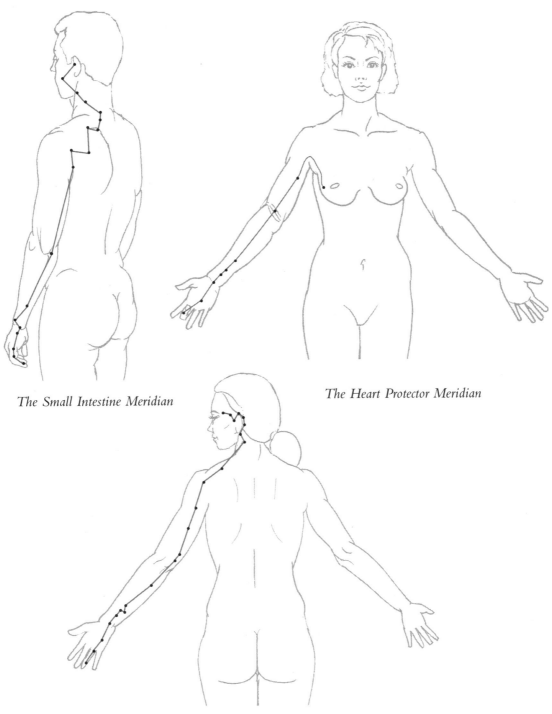

The Small Intestine Meridian

The Heart Protector Meridian

The Triple Heater Meridian

FIRE OUT OF BALANCE

When out of balance, Fire can become either excess or deficient, or a combination of the two.

Fire in Deficiency

When Fire is deficient, the body-mind-spirit lacks its upper range of activity. There may be signs of cold, of weakness, of lack of animation, or of the restless activity typical of deficient blood, which is unable to nourish and ground body processes.

Fire deficiencies can manifest with any one or more of the following symptoms:

* palpitations
* pale complexion
* restlessness
* weak or erratic pulses
* anxiety
* cold hands and feet
* no light in the eyes
* disturbed dreams
* insomnia
* lack of joy
* inability to follow through
* stuttering or difficulty speaking

Other symptoms may include numbness, dizziness, fatigue, inability to form or maintain close personal relationships, lack of effect, no vitality, aphasia, catatonia, poor concentration. Creatively, someone with deficient Fire begins many projects, but usually abandons them in midstream. The intense involvement required by the Fire phase to get something really going is too overwhelming to those with deficient Fire, so they abandon it and move on to something else.

Jim A. suffered from deficient Fire. His predominant physical symptoms included chest tightness, palpitations, and anxiety. Jim's hands were noticeably cold to the touch, and his manner when he spoke was joyless and complaining. He moved slowly, and was slow to take action and make decisions. Jim had no close friends, and would often use alcohol to "open himself up" around people—particularly women—which made him feel temporarily less frustrated and lonely, though he would later withdraw and become hostile toward the people he had thus opened himself up to. He could not maintain relationships in the face of the commitment they demanded of him. General trouble maintaining things was also evident in Jim's schooling—he had dropped out of college after a year, and nearly dropped out of professional school as well. When asked what he did for fun, Jim replied that he didn't know, then reported that he was "too busy" to have fun.

Jim's lack of Fire presented itself physically and emotionally. His inability to have fun, and his inability to connect with others in a meaningful way, point to Heart deficiency. His palpitations, anxiety, and tightness in the chest also indicate Heart issues. The fact that Jim moved and acted slowly reveals a lack of Fire's rapid and random movement, while dropping out of school—in this case— could be attributed to an inability to engage with Fire's "full throttle" energies.

My heart was split,
  and a flower
  appear'd,

and grace
  sprang up,

and it bore fruit
  for my God.

—Song of Solomon

When Fire deficiency is the main imbalance, the other elements are likely to displace as follows:

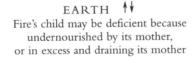

EARTH ↑↓
Fire's child may be deficient because
undernourished by its mother,
or in excess and draining its mother

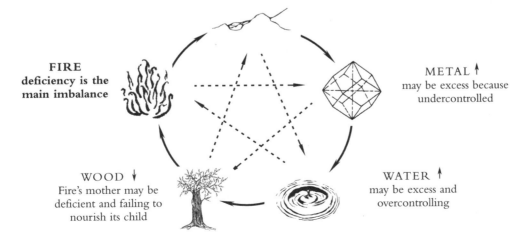

FIRE
deficiency is the
main imbalance

METAL ↑
may be excess because
undercontrolled

WOOD ↓
Fire's mother may be
deficient and failing to
nourish its child

WATER ↑
may be excess and
overcontrolling

*The supernatural
forces of summer
create heat
in the Heavens
and fire on Earth;
they create the
heart and the
pulse within
the body . . . the
red color, the
tongue, and the
ability to express
laughter . . .
they create the
bitter flavor,
and the emotions
of happiness
and joy.*

*—The Yellow
Emperor's Classic of
Internal Medicine*

Fire excess, on the other hand, manifests with behavior exactly opposite Jim's—overexcitement, overinvolvement, and commitment that promises more than can actually be achieved. Too much Fire can cause symptoms of heat, of stagnation, of excess activity, and of the spirit not rooted. Common symptoms of Fire excess include:

* palpitations
* flushed face
* ruddy or purplish complexion
* purplish lips
* pounding pulses
* infections or inflammation
* sleeplessness
* inappropriate laughter
* overtalking
* hyperactivity
* anxiety

Other symptoms may include attention deficit disorder, manic episodes, and mental illness.

Creatively, excess Fire types tend to engage in many projects simultaneously, bringing intense enthusiasm to all of them. However, because their Fire continuously revs them up, these people usually can't concentrate long enough on any one project to bring it to completion.

Julia J. came to acupuncture for relief from carpal tunnel syndrome (pain and numbness in the fingers and wrists).

Julia's pain ran straight up the Heart Protector meridian and continued along her upper back, following the Small Intestine meridian. She also suffered from anxiety and poor sleep. During her initial visit, Julia reported that her problems had begun a few days after she realized she was in love with her boyfriend. She speculated that she found this situation extremely frightening

False Fire

There is also a special category of combined Fire deficiency and excess known as "false Fire" or "false heat." In this pattern, people exhibit modified Fire signs, which are a result of a deficiency that makes heat signs visible though they are not actually excessive.

EARTH ↑↓
Fire's child may be
deficient because of energy
blockage or excess because
overflowed into

METAL ↓
may be deficient because
overcontrolled

FIRE
**excess is the
main imbalance**

WATER ↓
may be deficient and
undercontrolling

WOOD ↑
Fire's mother may be
excess and overflowing
into its child

because she normally liked to be in control of herself, but felt quite vulnerable in love. In this case, Julia's fears about love and trust overwhelmed her Heart Protector, which manifested an excess along its meridian and then spread to other Fire organs.

False Fire is a deficiency condition (of Yin and Water) marked by exhaustion and weakness.

False heat symptoms include:

★ flushed cheeks (not full face)

- ★ night sweats
- ★ mouth sores
- ★ feelings of heat in the palms and soles
- ★ fatigue
- ★ difficulty sleeping
- ★ late-afternoon fevers

Emotionally, someone with false heat might have similar behavior to one with a true excess, although they will seem more hysterical and, as a rule, will exhaust themselves quite quickly. Often, false heat develops from true excess Fire: Long-term Fire excess consumes the body's Yin, which thereafter fails to balance Fire's Yang.

FIRE AND ACUPUNCTURE

The meridians of the Heart, Small Intestine, Heart Protector, and Triple Heater carry Fire's energy throughout the body. Disturbances along these meridians may reflect Fire imbalances, which can be treated with acupuncture to improve or prevent chronic illness. When acupuncture is used to treat the Fire element, the points on the Fire meridians most commonly used are those that correspond to the Five Elements.

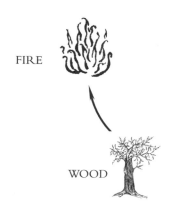

FIRE

WOOD

The **Wood** points on the Fire meridians treat Fire through its mother in the Creation cycle. They are often used to tonify Fire deficiencies.

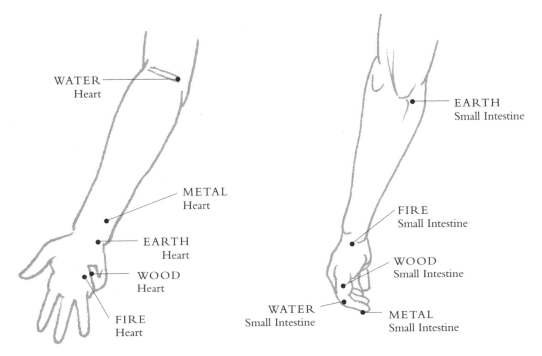

The Five Element Points on the
Heart Meridian

The Five Element Points on the
Small Intestine Meridian

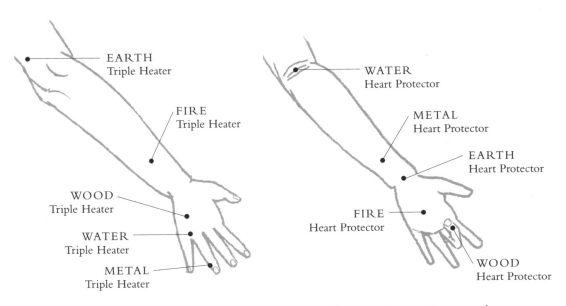

The Five Element Points on the
Triple Heater Meridian

The Five Element Points on the
Heart Protector Meridian

The **Fire** points on Fire meridians have a particularly powerful effect, and may be used whenever Fire energy needs to be adjusted—for instance, to tonify or reduce Fire itself, to tonify Earth, Fire's child, or to control Metal.

The **Metal** points on Fire meridians can be tonified when excess Fire is overcontrolling Metal, or dispersed to stop Metal from backing up into Fire.

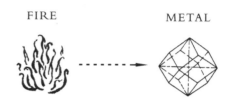

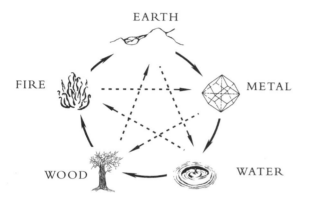

The **Water** points on the Fire meridians are commonly tonified to control excess Fire, and dispersed to prevent Water from overcontrolling Fire and causing deficiency.

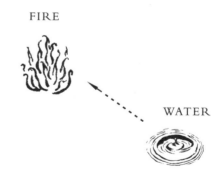

The **Earth** points on the Fire meridians are used to affect the relationship between Fire and Earth, its child. Children in the Creation cycle naturally draw energy from their mothers; the Earth points on the Fire meridians are thus commonly used to drain excess energy from Fire.

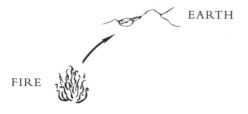

A treatment based on Five Element dynamics might treat a Fire excess with Water points to control Fire excess, and with Earth points to drain Fire excess through its child.

Julia J., described earlier, was treated with a combination of Fire and Water points—especially on her Heart Protector meridian where her carpal tunnel syndrome was most active. After the first treatment, her pain was significantly improved, and successive treatments eliminated the problem completely. Julia also reported that her anxiety diminished greatly, and she returned a few weeks before her marriage to calm her prewedding jitters.

For Fire deficiency, one might use Wood points to tonify Fire through its mother, while dispersing Water points to stop Water from overcontrolling.

Jim A. came for three acupuncture treatments, and felt that his anxiety was abating. The following week he broke up with his newest girlfriend and decided to discontinue treatments, however, saying that he "wasn't ready" to change his habits.

FIRE AND FOOD

The Fire element manifests in the foods we eat as the bitter flavor, as vegetables that branch outward, as fruits that grow around a central pit, and as the color red. The Fire element also governs foods with a warming thermal nature. Foods that are warming add heat—add Fire—to the body, and therefore share an affinity with the Yang elements of Wood and Fire.

Fire's flavor: bitter

Like the other flavors, bitterness aligns with the Five Element Control cycle, and has characteristics of Fire's controlling element, Water. Bitterness is Yin, cooling, and causes body energy to descend, and is therefore useful in dishes and diets meant to control excess Fire, or to tonify Water.

Because it is cooling, the bitter flavor clears excess heat or Fire; because it descends body energy, bitterness also drains dampness, moving it downward into the Bladder for elimination in the urine. In addition to the excess Fire conditions discussed earlier in this chapter, the bitter flavor is also quite useful for clearing Wood excesses, and those conditions that combine excesses of Wood and Fire.

Some examples of foods with bitter flavors are romaine lettuce, rye, alfalfa, watercress, bitter melon, dandelion greens, and aloe juice. Foods that are both bitter and pungent include citrus peels, scallions, turnips, and white pepper. Foods that are both bitter and sweet include amaranth, asparagus, celery, lettuce, papaya, and quinoa. Herbs with a bitter flavor, like gold-enseal and yellow dock, often make potent antibiotics, as their bitterness clears the heat of infection.

The bitter flavor penetrates the Heart and the Small Intestine, Fire's primary organs. It can therefore be added to diets of people who have Heart or Small Intestine disorders of any kind, although it should be used in moderation for cases of deficiency.

Fire's thermal nature: hot

All foods in Chinese medicine have a thermal nature that describes their effects on body energy. Fire's thermal nature is hot—hot foods add heat to body systems, increasing their overall activity and raising energy.

Some examples of warm or hot foods include ginger, cinnamon, cloves, basil, rosemary, oats, spelt, quinoa, sunflower and sesame seeds, walnuts, pine nuts, fennel, anise, caraway, carob, cumin, rice, corn, buckwheat, rye, parsnips, onions, cherries, pumpkin, basmati rice, citrus peels, hot peppers, cayenne, butter, anchovies, mussels, trout, chicken, beef, and lamb.

Because they add Fire, foods with a warm or hot thermal nature should be used in cases of Fire deficiency, and avoided during Fire excess.

Fire's vegetables: branching and spreading

Foods that spread outward as they grow also share an affinity with Fire, and can be used to tonify Fire in the diet. Leafy greens like spinach, kale, and broccoli all spread outward like Fire. However, these vegetables should be eaten cooked, not raw, and should be used in combination with more warming foods for Fire deficiencies.

Fire's fruits: pitted

Fruits that grow around a central pit like apricots, peaches, and cherries are also Fire foods. They are good for tonifying deficient fire but should be eaten in moderation, as they can have a cooling thermal nature.

Tonifying Fire Deficiency

Warming foods as described earlier are the most important part of any Fire tonification plan. The addition of sweet and pungent foods (see Earth and Metal chapters) can also help to warm the body and tonify Fire deficiencies.

Methods of preparation that require longer cooking times, like baking, frying, and roasting, also tonify Fire by imparting more heat to the food, which then carries it into the body.

Fire deficiency can occur during cold weather—in winter and also in autumn, when the body prepares for colder weather—and can also be generated internally at any time of year from overwork, long illness, or emotional causes. At these times, it's a good idea to adhere to a diet of hearty warming foods, larger portions, and more fats, oils, and meats. Warm teas, hot baths, and long-cooked stews and roasts are also appropriate, while salads, iced beverages, and dairy products should be avoided.

Many vegetarians develop internal Fire deficiencies because they don't have enough warming foods in their diets. Particularly in cold climates, the lack of meat's warm energy can contribute to symptoms like cold hands and feet, pale or grayish complexions, fatigue, depression, anxiety, nervousness, belching, abdominal pain, and constipation. Since many vegetarians also eat a lot of cooling foods like salads, raw vegetables, soy products, and dairy products like cheese and yogurt, they further damage the body's Fire. Although some people fare well on a vegetarian diet, it is not particularly balanced from a Chinese medical point of view, and, therefore, not widely recommended as a long-term habit. It can be useful, however, for short periods of time in cleansing and reducing Wood and Fire excesses.

1 leg of lamb, 7 to 8 lbs.

3 large cloves of garlic, slivered

2 tbsp. olive oil

1 tbsp. brown mustard

1 tbsp. water

2 tbsp. dried thyme leaves

2 tbsp. dried rosemary leaves

2 tsp. ground coriander seeds

2 tbsp. coarsely ground black pepper

fresh rosemary sprigs for garnish

1. Preheat oven to 425°F.
2. Cut slits all over lamb with a sharp knife and insert garlic slivers.
3. Brush lamb all over with olive oil.
4. Combine the mustard, water, thyme, rosemary, coriander seeds, and pepper in a small bowl and mix thoroughly. Put this mixture all over the lamb to form a crust.
5. Place in shallow roasting pan on center rack and cook for 45 minutes. Reduce heat to 375°F and cook for an additional 30 minutes.
6. Remove, rest loosely covered for 15 minutes. Carve, garnish with fresh rosemary, and serve. Serves 5.

Controlling Fire Excess: food and summer

Fire tends toward excess in summer, its season, but it can also become excess at any time of year due to stress, illness, or overwork.

Like all excess patterns in the Five Element cycle, excess Fire can be controlled most readily by eating foods associated with its flavor—bitterness. Whether Fire is excess internally, with the physical and emotional symptoms described above, or externally, because of summer temperatures, one's menu should be varied, with meals that are light and bright. Plenty of fruits and vegetables, bright colors, a small amount of spicy flavors, and, above all, a wide variety. Also include foods with a cooling thermal nature like cucumber, salad greens, watermelon, sprouts, lemons, and limes (see the Water chapter for a more complete list of cooling foods).

In summertime, vegetables can occasionally be eaten raw as salads—particularly by people who tend toward excess generally. For the most part, however, vegetables should be lightly steamed in order to prevent damage to the Spleen (see Earth chapter).

It is important to note that cooling in Chinese medicine is done with foods that have a cooling nature—not through frozen or chilled food and drink. These are considered neither healthy nor cooling; in fact, they cause the Stomach to create more heat in order to break the foods down, which ultimately damages the entire digestive system. Even in Western nutritional theory, cold beverages are not as cooling as room-temperature ones, because cold causes vessels to contract so that they don't absorb the liquid.

Moderate amounts of spices—like chili peppers, cayenne, and ginger—can be used to cool the body as well, although it can be a tricky business. According to Chinese medical theory, these warming foods can clear heat when used in moderation. For although they warm the body initially, their spreading nature pushes all the heat toward the body's surface, where it is released as sweat, which then cools the body. For the same reason, hot teas like mint and chamomile can be cooling. However, treating Fire excesses in this way can be complicated,

FIRE-DISPERSING RECIPE

Dandelion Greens and Dried Cherries with Raspberry Vinaigrette

These bitter greens are a perfect combination for reducing excess Fire and/or Wood.

Thoroughly wash two bunches of dandelion greens, then chop into 1-inch pieces. Steam them lightly, then toss with a handful of dried cherries or cranberries. To make the vinaigrette, combine ¼ cup of raspberry vinegar with ¼ cup of extra virgin olive oil and a pinch of salt. Dress the greens and enjoy with fish or another main dish.

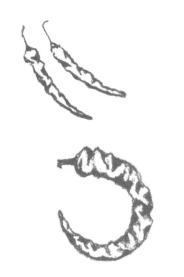

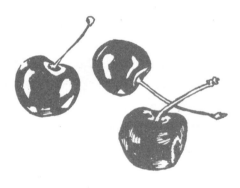

*Some examples of
Fire foods*

and can exacerbate the excess if done improperly or if sweating does not occur. It may be best to consult a Chinese medical nutritionist or herbalist before undertaking this strategy.

Foods to avoid in times of Fire excess are the heavy ones, like meats, eggs, and oils. They cause sluggishness and create internal heat. For additional ways to control excess Fire with food, tonify Water as described in the food section of the Water chapter.

FIRE AND QIGONG

The Fire element has a natural affinity with the Spirit, one of QiGong's Three Treasures. Called Shen in Chinese medicine, the spirit has a number of different manifestations. Because of this, many practitioners find it helpful to distinguish between a "Big Shen" and a "little shen." The "Big Shen" refers to Spirit in general and is an expression of the force of creation. It embodies peace, a sense of belonging, and a knowledge of the unity of all things. The proverbial "ghost in the machine," Shen is the true origin of all beings. It is the object of "spiritual" concerns, and the entity whose attributes are discussed throughout this book.

Little shen, on the other hand, refers to those aspects of spirit that are directly connected to the Heart and the Fire element. Whereas Big Shen involves the whole being and all the elements, little shen describes what the Heart gives: warmth, love, a sparkle in the eyes, and vitality in the body. It also refers to what we call the mind in Western culture, which is responsible for consciousness, awareness, and thought. Little shen is more easily disturbed by minor imbalances of the Heart and can cause symptoms like anxiety, disturbed sleep, or mania; Big Shen is disturbed by severe trauma and manifests its disturbances in serious mental illnesses.

In fact, however, Big Shen and little shen are really one and the same; they are simply different aspects of what we call spirit, which is housed in the Heart and is therefore a natural part of Fire's purview. The seeking and transcendent nature of the spirit shares Fire's qualities of raising, dispersing, and merging; it is ephemeral and has a tendency—like smoke—to dissipate. (People who are spiritually or intellectually oriented also tend to dissipate in this manner; absent-minded professors and New Age groupies often have trouble functioning in the world because they are continually floating above it.)

Because of its Fiery nature, the spirit requires cooling and grounding in order to keep it from dispersing. Meditation, which draws from the stillness and power of the Water element, is the perfect companion of spirit, nourishing its Fire with calmness and a sense of tranquillity. Disciplining the mind as movement disciplines the body, meditation allows us to release the worries and obstacles that block us from knowledge of our highest selves, while controlling the restless ascent of our intellects. As we meditate, we reconnect with a grounded spirit and rediscover our path.

Meditation is a mainstay of Eastern arts as well as most religious and shamanic traditions. It can take the form of ritual and directed prayer, or can be a simple exercise to quiet the mind. Connecting us with the heart of the universe, meditation stills our restless minds and joins us with the greater mind—the universal source of compassion and peace. Meditation is a doorway through which we access the greater universe, where we release our individual egos to remember what it is like to feel unalone.

Meditation thus affords us a different perspective on our lives and our difficulties. It returns us to a place of peace and no judgment, from which we are better able to take appropriate action. While meditation can be practiced sitting, standing, lying down, or walking, the sitting meditation described below is a good way to begin.

Meditation can also be combined with visualization and breathing practices to effect healing in the body. Energy can be directed through the breath and vision to any places of tension or disease, or healing thoughts can be directed toward others. We can ask for guidance from the universe,

MEDITATION

Sit comfortably on a small, firm cushion or against a wall. Close the eyes and breathe deeply and slowly three times, being sure to exhale fully each time. Notice any areas of tension in the body and try to let them relax. Then turn your attention to the breath. Feel your body inhaling and exhaling and try to visualize your body filling up with fresh qi and exhaling stale qi with each breath. Do this for three or four breaths. Try to feel your thoughts coming and going as freely as your breath. Don't obsess or attach to any particular one, but pay attention to them as carefully as if you watched each breath, letting them come and go at their own speed. As disturbing or repetitive thoughts come through, they may quicken or disrupt the breath, or create tension in the body. If this happens, make a point of slowing down and relaxing, of honoring the thought while disengaging from its disturbing power. After a few minutes, your thoughts should be slower and calmer. Try to keep your attention focused on them rather than wandering off into fantasy or sleep. You may choose at this time to focus on certain body parts, trying to visualize but not control their activities. After about fifteen minutes, bring your attention back to the breath. Gently quicken it, and start to wiggle your hands and feet in preparation for waking up. As you come back into your body, slowly open your eyes, while concentrating on the sense of inner peace and calm now evident. When you stand up, you should feel rested, relaxed, and peaceful.

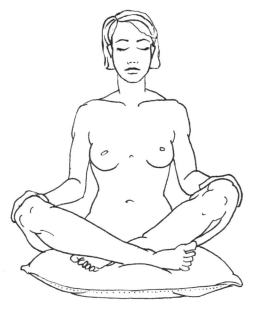

Meditation

wisdom, healing, and strength. Because meditation connects us to our source, we can use this time to reaffirm our purpose and to redirect ourselves toward it.

FIRE AND FENG SHUI

In our indoor and outdoor environments, Fire bursts forth in the color red, in sunlight or any kind of light, in electricity, in flames or fire, in furnaces and radiators, and in sharp corners and sharp peaks.

Outdoors, the Fire element is invoked everywhere the sun shines. The sun's light, heat, and expansive energy make it a hallmark of the Fire element, and a perennial Yang symbol. In cloudy climates and darker seasons Fire is therefore often deficient, while summertime and latitudes near the Equator are characterized by excess Fire. The summer solstice, when earth experiences its longest period of sunlight, is often celebrated with bonfires, all-night parties, music, and dancing—activities that celebrate the Fire element's movement and joy.

Lights can be used to stimulate Fire outdoors, brightening paths to the house, driveways, and any areas of excess darkness or Yin. They can also be used to "cure" ill-shaped plots of land or poorly placed buildings. For instance, an L-shaped building, normally regarded as unstable because of the missing piece, can be harmonized with the addition of a light in the absent quarter.*

Pointy or craggy rock formations and mountain peaks correspond with Fire. In classical Feng Shui, such formations are considered to have unstable energy—like Fire—and are therefore not suitable sites for homes or businesses. Tall and pointed buildings

* Sarah Rossbach, *Interior Design with Feng Shui.*

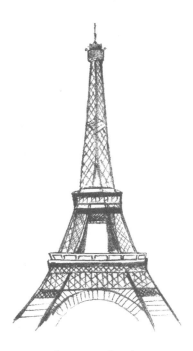

The triangular shape and pointed top of the Eiffel Tower identify it as a Fire structure.

like the Empire State Building also correspond to Fire.

Indoors, red is the color of Fire and heat. Wherever it appears, red warms and stimulates the eye and the Heart. Red ribbons are a classical Feng Shui cure for any kind of imbalance, and can be hung wherever energy needs to be stimulated (according to the Ba-Gua, for instance).

Pink and peach are good colors for the master bedroom—or the room of someone who wishes to get married—as they promote Fire's warming love. In addition, red bricks and terra-cotta can be warming, fiery influences in a home. As mixtures of Earth and Fire, these materials add warmth without the over-the-top intensity of brighter reds.

In the home, Fire *shapes* rise to a point, like corners, candles, and triangles. Sometimes Wood and Fire are closely blended in an object, making it difficult to separate the two. Standing lamps, for instance, with lightbulbs at the top have a definite Fire aspect to them (the light itself), though the general shape may be more like Wood. In general, Fire shapes are thinner and sharper.

Because Fire is unstable, sharp corners and sharp tools are considered dangerous, and should not point out into rooms, toward chairs or beds, or other places where people might be injured by an aggressive "arrow" of energy. Red ribbons hung on such corners, or mirrors hung so as to reflect them back on themselves, can ameliorate their dangerous effects.

Fire *colors* are red and pink and bright orange.

Fire *materials* are anything that conducts light, heat, or fire—lightbulbs, heating vents, stoves—particularly gas stoves, which have a pilot always lit.

Stoves are particularly important in classical Feng Shui, as they represent a source of both warmth and food. They are closely associated with prosperity, and should therefore be kept clean and used often. The burners are particularly important; they should be used equally, and a mirror can be placed at the back of the stove so as to give the appearance of more of them.

The Fire area of the Ba-Gua is the southern wall of a room or home. This area also corresponds to fame. To tonify a deficient Fire element in your life, or to encourage your fame or rank, hang a red ribbon or other red decoration on the south wall of the living room, bedroom, kitchen, or study.

The southwest corner of a room corresponds to marriage, and can be stimulated with ribbons, lights, or colored mobiles to invite a new marriage or to harmonize an existing one. These adjustments will be most effective when applied to a bedroom.

The three months of summer denote prosperity and abundance. Heaven and earth exchange their influences; the ten thousand things appear in all their splendor and ripeness. Man goes to bed at night and rises early. He strives for consummate radiance and causes his own influences to flow away, as if that which he loves lies outside of himself.

—The Yellow Emperor's Classic of Internal Medicine

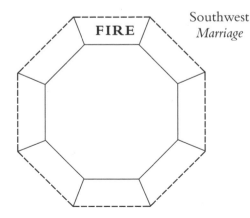

South
Fame/Rank

FIRE

Southwest
Marriage

Tonifying Fire Deficiency

If you're feeling gloomy and in need of some joy, try wearing something red—socks, underwear, mittens, tie, etc. Bring home some red pillows or fresh flowers and create a "Fire corner," where you can go to charge up. Paint a small shelf or window frame a nice shade of red. Buy a box of red candles and place them around the house in attractive holders. Remember, though, that Fire's energy has a tendency to rage out of control—so work with it carefully. Keep it in small doses, and experiment with pink or rose if red seems too intense. In addition, create or buy some angular art, spend an afternoon painting triangles and fires. Look around your house and focus on those things that are pointy, angled, and rising. Add a new lamp to a dark corner, and replace dim lightbulbs with brighter ones.* Light candles, build a fire if you have a fireplace, look at pictures of hot, sunny places and of your summer vacations of the past.

For other ways of tonifying Fire, tonify Wood and reduce Water as instructed in those chapters.

Dispersing Fire Excess

For Fire excess, it is best to limit the amounts of light, heat, sharpness, and red color in your home and wardrobe. Western windows might be oppressive with their harsh afternoon light; hang a crystal or a prism to disperse it. Also see the Water chapter for information on how to tonify Water in order to control Fire, and tonify Earth to help drain Fire's excess through its child.

---

* It is a good idea to use full-spectrum bulbs (like those manufactured by Chromalux), or those made for plants. These have spectral energies more like sunlight and are healthier for the body. They are also helpful for those who suffer from seasonal affective disorder (SAD) brought on by lack of sunlight.

When the Fire element is in healthy balance, our relationships with others have a smooth and measured flow: Trust builds steadily, love comes easily, and we are not surprised by too much confusion or hurt because we protect ourselves appropriately from those who have not yet proven themselves reliable. Healthy Fire gives us the capacity for joy and the enthusiasm to fulfill our goals, the desire to reach out and the faith that we will find what we seek. Above all, Fire gives us a warm and steady zest for life—as strong and as regular as the heartbeat that circulates our blood.

With its consuming reach and frenetic energy, Fire illuminates the edges of reality. It suggests what is highest, farthest, hottest, and most intense about the experience of living. At Fire's edge we are more alive, and more aware of every thought, emotion, and sensation. The gift of Fire surrounds our peak experiences—creating the moments that elevate and transform us forever.

When Fire has played itself out, however, it leaves gray ash in its aftermath and nothing more. Though it looks drab and insignificant, if we were to disregard this ash we would be failing to learn the real lessons of Fire. In fact, ash is everything: It is so rich in minerals that it fertilizes ground for centuries to come. Volcanic lava and its ash form the base of new land masses that nourish seeds and civilizations alike. The ash that drifts to ground after a fire *becomes* ground, becomes Earth, becomes the matrix that nourishes all. Earth is Fire's child, formed in the beauty and intensity of Fire's storm. It is the solidness and reality that still exist when Fire's headiness has vaporized everything else. It is the nourishing medium that gives birth to the phoenix, who rises from Fire's ashes to begin life anew.

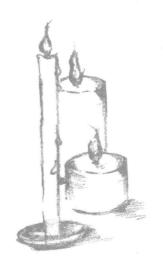

EARTH

EARTH IS THE MOTHER OF LIFE. WITH ITS OFFSPRING
of grasses and trees, animals and people, insects, waters, foods,
and eaters, the Earth has been a figure of worship since the
earliest times. A source of mystery and a focus of human
survival, the Earth and its vicissitudes form the basis of many
of the world's religions. Because Earth's fertility is so strongly
associated with female fecundity, the Earth depicted in many
mythologies is a female character, and, more specifically, a
mother. To the Greeks she was Gaia, to the early Danes
Nerthus, to the Hindus Durga or Shakti, to Native Americans
simply our Mother. Around the world, Earth is the mother
and continuing nurturer of life.

Though primarily nurturing, many Earth figures react
with rage when betrayed or otherwise angered—droughts,
fires, earthquakes, and floods are some of the weapons at their
disposal. In this role she is both creator and destroyer—
a duality conspicuously plain in tales of the Hindu Kali, who

is responsible for destroying that which she creates, and in the crone figure of feminine spirituality movements—an old woman who appears as a harbinger of death.

Many creation epics describe a sacred marriage between the feminine Earth and the masculine Sky, who thus create the earth's creatures. The Greek Gaia and Ouranos created time, the Earth, the mountains, the gods, and people. China's Yin Earth and Yang Heavens joined forces to create humankind, while Native Americans' Mother Earth and Father Sky created Brother Sun and Sister Moon and all else that followed. Although monotheistic religions have few overt feminine aspects of divinity (the Virgin Mary being an exception), the Old Testament's Adam—the first man—was formed by God out of "clay" or "earth"—a symbol of the feminine.

Though essentially feminine, the Earth element of the Five Element cycle is not overtly a creator or a destroyer. Rather, it is a matrix that contains, allows, and supports living processes, as well as a fulcrum around which the other elements turn. Like the growth medium in a petri dish, or the grid on which a graph is plotted, Earth is a medium in which everything else happens. It is passive and receptive, defining the space in which matter exists.

In the Creation cycle, Earth is created by Fire, whose ash represents something new and raw when all else has burned away. Like volcanic ash or forest fire ash, the remains of fire are spectacularly nurturing to new growth. In the Control cycle, Earth

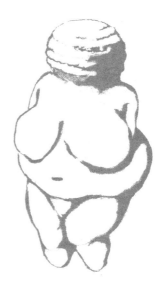

Earth-goddess figures like the Venus of Willendorf (above), and the Seated Goddess from Catal Hayuk (below), embody many Earth-element characteristics: abundance, nurturing, and the feminine principle.

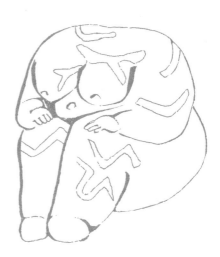

is controlled by Wood, whose aggressive growth puts boundaries on Earth's ability to give.

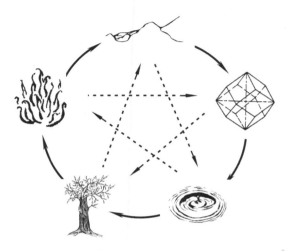

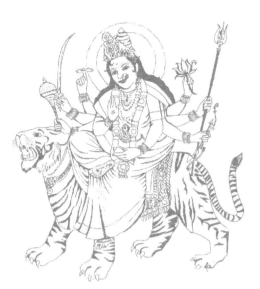

The Hindu mother-
goddess, Durga, is the
goddess of rulers
and warriors, a giver
of prosperity, and
the dispenser of food
to humankind.

As the center of the Five Element cycle, Earth is considered the prime stabilizing force. Whereas energy expands throughout the Wood and Fire phases, and contracts through Metal and Water, Earth is that point in the middle where there is transition and a carefully mediated balance that controls it. Earth's centering forces are present wherever transition occurs, so that in the Five Element cycle—whose very essence is about change—Earth presides over continuity. In a sense, Earth is the home of all the elements, and the stable center in which they are grounded. While each of the elements contains aspects of all the others (see "Origin" on page 2), Earth more than any of them reflects the whole of the cycle, and can be defined in terms of it. Earth's attributes can be understood as its Wood, Fire, Earth, Metal, and Water aspects.

1. EARTH'S WOOD
Contains

Earth sets boundaries that contain and define activities, processes, and events. Like the trunk of a tree that delimits it as an individual organism, this aspect of Earth energy delimits borders. Not of individuals, but of spaces: Containment is defined by the space it creates within. A bottle, a room, office hours, laws—anything that holds, surrounds, or limits anything else relies upon the containment energies of the Earth element.

When containment defines and protects boundaries, it also protects that which is contained. Earth is thus a vessel that protects life as it would a liquid, which would otherwise be dispersed.

In the construction of a building, the containment aspect of the Earth element comes into play as soon as the building is habitable. When the roof and walls are in place, a building becomes a space for containing inhabitants, objects, businesses, or stored goods. This kind of containment embraces physical space, giving boundaries and shelter to whatever lies within.

Because the ultimate purpose of any construction is the creation of a container of one kind or another, an ethos of Earth energy governs all construction. By this token, all buildings, spaces, and vessels are predominantly Earth; every home, office, nest, tree hollow, and cave is a manifestation of the Earth element, as are bottles, jars, cups, chairs, and sofas because they surround and support something else. Because it demarcates lines that separate and define, containment is the Wood within the Earth phase.

2. EARTH'S FIRE
Balances

During the Earth phase of a cycle, primal energies balance and change direction. When opposing energies (like Yang and Yin) shift dominance, Earth controls the smoothness of their transition. On a physical level, Earth balances potential and kinetic energies; like the fulcrum of a lever, it holds the center and allows the balance of energies to shift.

A complicated concept, balance is not just stillness, but the management of opposing forces. If you try balancing

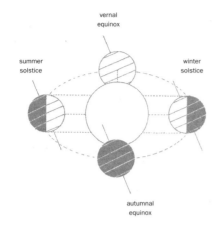

vernal
equinox

summer
solstice

winter
solstice

autumnal
equinox

The equinoxes and solstices represent points of transition, when the balance between sunlight and darkness changes.

on one foot while holding the other foot in your hands, you will wobble, and be forced to adjust yourself continually in an effort to maintain balance. There are hundreds of forces pulling in all directions at once, and balance is achieved only by accommodating them all.

The Earth element collects these conflicting forces and distributes them appropriately, maintaining balance in a given system. Whereas chaos would break it down, Earth element's ordered disbursement is the glue that holds any system together.

As a season, Earth corresponds to late summer and to the time of transition between each season—the days surrounding the equinoxes and solstices. At these times, the forces of daylight (Yang) and darkness (Yin) are uniquely balanced. In this capacity, Earth presides over the shifting connections of time, space, and relationship. In this regard, Earth is also considered to hold the center of the Five Element circle.

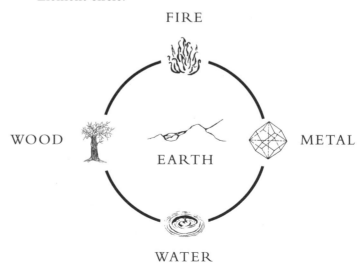

FIRE

WOOD

EARTH

METAL

WATER

The Earth phase of a day is the between-times—in particular, the meal-times that transition between morning and afternoon, and between afternoon and evening. This kind of transition, like the one between seasons, is a smoothly flowing one, occurring as Yin and Yang shift dominance. Note, however, that this is not the same as the absolute transformation that occurs during a real Fire phase; in the Fire phase, Yang reaches a point of maximal energy and vaporizes or merges with something else. In the transition characteristic of the Earth phase, however, nothing is maximizing—change happens in incre-ments as Yang slowly gives over to Yin, or vice versa. Earth balances and pre-sides over this incremental changing of the guard, but it is the flavor of merging and transformation that identifies bal-ance as the Fire of Earth.

On a cosmological level, Earth represents that point in evolution when the planet Earth, and the solar system around it, became self-regulating systems. As the early universe cooled, its rapid-fire evolution slowed and stabilized. With less development, individual life-forms on the planet Earth became more stable, as did the relationships between them.

They evolved to a state of homeostasis—a complex but essentially stable balance that permitted the ecosystem to grow without collapsing into chaos. Similarly, the planets in the solar system evolved their characteristic orbits, which reflect the stable gravitational relationships each planet has with all the others.

Homeostasis reflects a merging of many forces into a functional and stable whole. The delicate balances and transitions that are required to main-tain such a state are firmly grounded in Earth's fiery energies.

3. EARTH'S EARTH
Accumulates

As an element, Earth is the soil that collects and contains nutrients and moisture, keeping them available for seeds and roots to draw from. Earth accumulates by collecting resources that can be stored and disbursed at an appropriate time. In this sense soil is a medium in which growth can occur; though itself neither a growing thing nor a nutrient, soil contains and fosters both. This quality of collecting and accumulating is Earth's Earth. (Note also that soil is composed of many different ingredients, including the decayed remnants of dead plants and animals. Here, Earth acts as a transition point between death and rebirth, recycling dead plants and animals into a medium that nourishes new growth.)

A squirrel's yearly gathering of nuts is classic Earth behavior, as is the pooling and puddling of water in rain barrels and troughs. People who collect things—whether stamps, items with a frog theme, or great artworks—similarly demonstrate Earth's acquisitiveness. Accumulation creates stores of resources that can (ideally) be used at a future time. Clay vessels produced around the world epitomize this function—jars, pots, and bowls have carried and stored our food resources since time immemorial.

Anything to do with food or eating involves the Earth element's faculties of collection; eating epitomizes the gathering of resources. As we take food into

ABOUT CLAY

Clay is a variant of soil that epitomizes many Earth functions. Its round-bellied bowls, jars, and pots—used as containers even today—evoke the image of the round and pregnant mother that the Earth element represents; even the earliest clay sculptures depict big-breasted and wide-hipped icons of the great fertile mother. Infinitely moldable, clay embodies the Earth element's flexibility and receptivity. The very molecules of clay, arranged in perfect crystals, have more surface area than any other known material, which allows them to reach and react with what's around them quite thoroughly. Used medicinally to draw impurities out of the body, used domestically to create bowls and pots as well as bricks for building, and used artistically for sculpture, clay is one of the most versatile materials known. Some biologists even believe that clay was the ingredient that first allowed organic life to be created from inorganic matter—making it the mother of all life indeed.

our bodies, we collect the bulk and the nutrients of the planet within ourselves, transforming it into fuel as needed. Money is also an Earth element phenomenon that illustrates Earth's accumulative nature. Although the gold standard itself is governed by Metal, our exchanges of it involve the same gathering and giving that we apply to nutrients and every other resource.

4. EARTH'S METAL
Nurtures

Another aspect of Earth's energy is the disbursement of the resources it collects. Vital to every process of reproduction, Earth nurtures by giving of itself to foster new life. In the life cycle of a tree, for instance, the nutrient-dense fruit (which doesn't support itself, but draws nutrients from the leaves) represents a sort of *donation* by the tree of its resources, which will be used in the propagation of a new tree. Earth nurtures like any mother suckling her young—by giving away parts of herself to ensure the young one's continued growth. This giving, however, does not come without a price; the resources donated are lost to the mother, often draining her in the process. While less painful than the Metal element's out-and-out loss, nurturing echoes its theme, and is therefore considered Earth's Metal aspect.

All reproduction is, similarly, an Earth element phenomenon, as are child-rearing, farming, gardening, and other activities that involve taking care

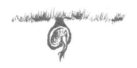

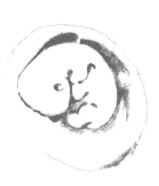

of others. Many people nurture their businesses as well, particularly at the beginning, when so many resources are put in with little security of return. This generosity defines true nurturing—it does not expect anything in return.

In the menstrual cycle, Earth element governs days fifteen to twenty-one, called the secretory stage of the cycle. During this time, rising hormone levels cause glands to release nutrients into the uterus. These nutrients, drawn from the woman's body, will sustain a developing embryo, if there is one. This part of the menstrual cycle illustrates Earth's nurturing, as it involves the giving away of some parts of the whole to propagate new life.

5. EARTH'S WATER
Allows

The Earth element creates space for new lives to develop. Hollows in the ground and wombs in the female bodies show Earth's yielding qualities.

In the natural world, the Earth element is the matrix in which everything else happens—where the animal, vegetable, and mineral kingdoms make their home. In essence, Earth allows these forms to develop by creating a space in which they can grow. Not only a container, Earth fosters growth by hollowing space out of its own being, as in the holes we dig to plant trees in. Earth not only contributes her own resources, but also redefines her own boundaries in order to include and allow other lives to take shape.

The space Earth creates is like a womb that stretches to accommodate the growing offspring within—it is generous and boundless, allowing whatever is needed. This inner space is like the undifferentiated unity of the Water element; from it new lives and ideas will take form. Though a full Water phase involves no strictures at all (see the Water chapter), Water within Earth creates space within boundaries. This tendency to create and allow space can be thought of as Earth's Water.

In creative (rather than procreative) processes, Earth is the time and space in which we allow ourselves to *be* creative. It is the room or the area in which we do creative work, and the time we allow for doing it. It is also our appreciation of the tools and the processes involved in the endeavor. Earth's generous allowance does not call for time frames or goals—it simply hollows out a space for us to do what we will. Though this will likely include some period of sitting and staring, or daydreaming, a stable Earth element does not lose patience or make demands, it simply holds the space. Only an environment that lets things percolate in this way will be fertile enough to sprout an exciting idea.

The totality of Earth's containing, balancing, accumulating, nurturing, and allowing properties is more than the sum of its parts; Earth as a whole is the very foundation of life, and its continuing source of nourishment and vitality. Because of its essential position at the center of the Five Element cycle, many consider Earth to be the most important element. A line of practitioners dating back to a fifth-century tradition known as the "Earth school" described most diseases as originating from imbalances in the Earth element, and most cures as being effected through it. Their saying "earth feeds all" describes the notion that Earth's transformations nourish all the other elements.

Tung Chung-Shu, a philosopher who lived in the second century B.C.E., described the Earth element in following manner:

> *Earth occupies the center, and is*
> *called the heavenly fructifier.*
> *It is the assister of Heaven. Its*
> *power is abundant and good,*
> *and cannot be assigned to the*
> *affairs of a single season only.*
> *Therefore among the five elements*
> *and four seasons, earth embraces*
> *all. Although metal, wood, water,*
> *and fire each have their own*

particular duties, they could not stand
were it not for earth. *

In a sense, the growing environmental movement is a sign of humanity's recognition of the centrality of Earth. Though the global ecological illness we now face is a result of our neglect of the Earth element's passive virtues, the current emphasis on "saving" the earth is a dramatic representation of our human culture struggling to honor its center—to honor the Earth element and all it represents.

The mysterious forces of the
Earth create moisture in the Heaven and
fertile soil upon the Earth; they create
the flesh within the body and the stomach
[and spleen]. They create the yellow
color . . . and give the voice the
ability to sing . . . they create the mouth,
the sweet flavor, and the emotions
of anxiety and worry.

—*The Yellow Emperor's Classic of Internal Medicine*

The Earth element renders itself climatically as dampness. Dampness describes moisture—not water itself, but the atmosphere of water and the rich particles suspended within it. It is the damp quality of good soil that surrounds roots with nutrients and

* Fung Yu-Lan, *A History of Chinese Philosophy, Vol. II.*

water, the dampness of clay, that makes it malleable, and air's "dampness" that makes it rich with the molecules that living things need to survive. Ripe fruits and vegetables are similarly damp (or moist) with their flavors and fragrances. Dampness in its proper measure surrounds and nourishes.

Physically, dampness is felt most acutely on humid days; it's an accumulation without which our tissues, skin, and muscles could not remain supple. Although moisture is most apparent on the outside of our bodies in humid weather—as the sweat on our skins—it lies beneath the skin in all weathers, lending ripeness and lusciousness to our flesh as it does to fruit.

Too much dampness, though, leads to rot—an overabundance of ripeness that leads to overripeness when it is not consumed. Rotting food, foul breath, and decomposing garbage are all examples of overaccumulations of dampness. Such overaccumulation in the body leads to feelings of heaviness and sluggishness in the limbs or head. Because moisture is heavy with nutrients, we feel burdened when it oversaturates us.

Dampness in the body also affects digestion and overall energy levels. In addition to the heaviness described above, many digestive problems such as gas and sluggish stool are symptoms of dampness, as is a lack of appetite, indecision about what to eat, or an inability to enjoy food. Phlegm, too, is a sign of dampness—it is moisture that has accumulated and condensed over a long period of time. Excess dampness in the mind leads to a foggy feeling and an inability to concentrate.

Dampness on another level is clutter. Too many items sitting around unused or underused accumulate dampness. Those who live in a constant state of physical dampness often live in cluttered spaces as well—they accumulate "stuff" around them on physical, emotional, and environmental levels.

Jenny and Al are a good-natured couple, kind and extremely nurturing toward others. They surround themselves with an abundance that reflects their generosity and their capacity to accumulate, but clutter certainly prevails over order in their home. Scarcely a day goes by that one of them doesn't bring some new toy or tool or piece of clothing into the house, where it gets piled on top of everything else. Even their refrigerator is crammed to the gills with food—half of it hidden from sight and rotting away, as is typical of an overabundant Earth element. Both suffer from chronic sinus conditions, and Al has a lot of respiratory phlegm as well, indicating over-dampness in the body as well as in the home.

On an emotional level, Earth's moisture manifests as caring, which draws upon its protective, nurturing, and accumulating energies. Like damp-ness, caring involves a certain amount of attention, of clinging to, of surrounding. When we care about somebody (or something), we give a portion of ourselves to them; our attention abides with them seeking comfort, safety, and nourishment on their behalf. Such caring nourishes like a rich soil, feeding the soul of those on whom it is bestowed.

Overcaring, though, leads to worry—the emotion associated with Earth in classical Chinese medicine. Worry brings the force of attention to bear too strongly on its object, not leaving enough room for it to grow naturally. Like overwatering a plant or overprotecting a child, worry interferes with what is none of its business. Where Earth in balance simply "allows" matters to transpire as they will, off balance it clings and festers, surrounding its object with imagined scenarios of danger and difficulty, thereby spoiling its true potential. In extreme cases, worry becomes obsession—a habit of clinging to the same unproductive thoughts over and over again.

In relationships, Earth energy governs emotional attachment. Whereas Fire pushes us to connect with

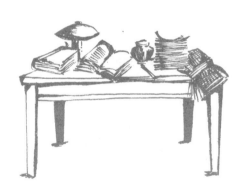

Clutter is an Earth-element imbalance that displays overabundance and a lack of containment.

others and opens a path of trust that allows us to do so, Earth defines and reinforces those connections over time. Earth bonds are built as people share experiences; this is the only way to become truly familiar with another human being. Earth bonds therefore attach slowly and meaningfully, and cannot be hurried, growing deeper in exact concordance with the level of shared history. Unlike a Fire connection that merges self with others completely for an instant, Earth bonds create a love that grows deeper and stronger with time.

Bonding is not simply emotional, however, it's also material. Strands of our essence lodge inside those we're bonded to, and vice versa, entwining our essential matrix with theirs. This interweaving alters our internal structures, and thus has the potential to distort or damage us if those whom we entrust act selfishly or manipulatively.

When people exchange gifts, they make the Earth bonds between them materially visible. We invest the gifts we give with our Earth energies, and *use* them, in a sense, to create or confirm the kinds of bonds we want. To people we don't know very well we are

likely to give gifts that don't require much knowledge of their tastes or personality—a bottle of wine or a bouquet of flowers, for instance, while we might exchange books, music, or personal items with friends we know a bit better.

With close friends, with family, and with lovers, we exchange still other kinds of gifts—jewelry, clothing, artwork, and similar things that tend to be more expensive and more personally tailored. And with spouses, long-term partners, or our children, we exchange expensive and intimate items like perfume, fancy jewelry, and vacations. As these gifts represent a deep level of connection and large sums of Earth-element time and money, they can occur only in the most intimate relationships.

Because they are invested with so much meaning, most people are highly sensitive to the hidden significance of gifts they receive. Katie B. became depressed when her boyfriend gave her a book about hiking for her birthday. She was disconsolate at the lack of intimacy the book portended, and figured (correctly) that the relationship was essentially over. Carla S. had a habit of unconsciously testing her relationships by knitting sweaters; she knew that an uncommitted partner would break up with her if she gave a sweater he was not ready to receive. In both of these cases, the givers invested gifts with the full weight of their Earth bonds, while those who received gifts were able to read in them the intentions of the giver.

EARTH IN THE HUMAN LIFE CYCLE

In the human life cycle, the Earth phase corresponds to the middle years—a time of stabilization and the creation of home, family, livelihood, and community. Ideally, this is a time of maturity, when we become fully independent and responsible for an Earth element that is capable of nurturing others as well as ourselves. And as we develop our own strong centers, we can also expand more fully into the outer world, becoming members of our community, our culture, and our planet.

In the creation of a home, we call upon Earth energies to give us shelter and protection. We create a kind of womb, surrounding ourselves with what comforts us, nurtures us, and protects us. Whether owned or rented, individual or shared, our homes restore us to safety and a sense of balance.

In creating a family, we explore the emotional bonds that the Earth element governs. Whether we have a partner, children, pets, and/or a family of friends, the people we surround ourselves with become the family with whom we play out our most intimate dramas. We learn to nurture and be nurtured, to love and be loved, refining the Earth element functions that we need for our own survival, and taking responsibility for the survival of others. At this stage we become figurative and literal parents who nurture new life into being.

In establishing a livelihood, we bring our unique selves into the world, sharing our time and talents in exchange for Earth element's money. It is an interchange that is characteristic of the Earth element, allowing resources to come in and flow out.

The making or joining of community further expands this interchange of self and world. As our home—our womb—becomes larger than our immediate environment, our bonds stretch to include a larger definition of self and relatedness. We begin to see ourselves as part of a human family, and, ideally, as part of a universal family.

In the development of the spirit, the Earth element governs centering, which is the ability to attune oneself to one's own presence. It clears our mental and emotional attention of distractions, allowing us to perceive our own thoughts and feelings accurately. Centering gives us the ability to concentrate and the power to react. Like the tone of a pure bell, centering allows us to resonate clearly with our own intent.

When our spirits are off center, it's like static interfering with a signal: What ought to be clear and strong becomes indiscernible. We find ourselves muddled, unable to concentrate, to think clearly, or even to figure out how we feel. When we are off center, we are absorbed in private noise instead of being in tune with the world around us. We lose contact with, and coherence in, the reality of the present.

In the activity of the soul, Earth corresponds to grounding. Grounding sinks energy downward, anchoring it in something stable. We can be grounded in our bodies, in the body of the earth, or in reality. Essentially these three are the same; they indicate contact with something real and immediate. On a physical level, grounding is like the solid and indisputable string that keeps a kite from flying out of control. Electrically, a grounded

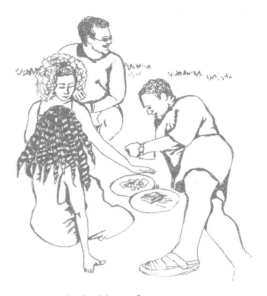

The building of community is an Earth-phase activity that sustains feelings of rootedness and belonging.

wire routes electricity into the earth so that it doesn't charge wild. When we are grounded internally, our imaginations are anchored to a sane reality. We are able to communicate with others because we have a stable reality in common with them.

When a soul is well grounded, it keeps the spirit from getting carried away; when a person is well grounded he is highly functional in the world, not "spaced out," or in a dream world—though he may certainly entertain hopes and dreams in private moments. In contrast, people who are not well grounded often seem to participate in a different reality entirely. They may be absorbed in worlds of fantasy, intellectual abstractions, or spiritual or emotional feelings; in contrast, their day-to-day needs will seem mundane and unappealing to them.

Jean Z. had a deficient Earth element and was never quite grounded. She often forgot things, and joked about how "spacey" she could be. With an unusually high and airy-sounding voice, she sounded spacey too. Jean worked only occasionally, and was supported by her boyfriend, whom she lived with. She had a lot of fantasies about wonderful, high-paying jobs as a model or a designer, but these never materialized. Not mean-spirited or untalented, Jean just lived in a different reality, one not bound by the exigencies of modern life. As she was not grounded enough to manage the hard work and minutiae of everyday living, Jean was largely dependent on other people's generosity for her survival.

Whereas work and self-discipline could have grounded her, Jean consistently made choices that further dissociated her from reality, like turning down work opportunities and continuing to focus on her fantasies of romance and riches. Jean's body, however, tried valiantly to anchor her: Her legs and buttocks were large and heavy, and she was often constipated. This combination revealed a whole lower body—including the stool—solidifying and putting on weight in an effort to pull Jean's energy earthward. She also had continual trouble with phlegm—a dense accumulation that often signals a body seeking solid ground.

EARTH IN THE BODY

The Earth element manifests in the body through the organs and meridians of the Spleen (Yin) and the Stomach (Yang). The Spleen and Stomach organs govern all Earth functions of bonding, nurturing, grounding, etc. They also preside over the following physical functions:

The Spleen governs digestion and absorption. Earth's accumulation and disbursement functions translate physically into the digestion and absorption of food. Specifically, the Spleen digests foods and fluids by extracting and refining their essences. It transports refined essences to the other Yin organs while sending impure essences toward the Yang organs of elimination.

The failure of these transformative functions creates dampness and phlegm, and can lead to generalized symptoms of deficiency and/or stagnation.

The Spleen builds Blood and qi. Like a nurturing mother, the Spleen contributes its richest products to the continued sustenance of the body. It helps to create both Blood and qi, the primary sources of energy and well-being. The Spleen contributes refined food essences to the Heart for production of Blood, and to the Lung and Kidneys for production of various forms of qi.

Imbalances in this aspect of Spleen function will lead to deficiencies of qi and/or Blood.

The Spleen directs ascending movements and holds things up. The Spleen directs the movement of those fluids and essences whose proper direction (according to Chinese physiology) is to move up—moving qi from the Spleen to the Lungs, for instance. It also holds the organs and blood vessels in their proper places, preventing confusion and collapse.

Dysfunctions in this aspect of the Spleen can lead to phlegm, diarrhea, or asthma, or to organ prolapses, varicose veins, and hemorrhoids.

The Spleen controls the flesh and holds things in place. An elastic yet strong container, flesh keeps our insides in. The Spleen determines overall shape and body type, and governs the health of the flesh. Overweight and underweight conditions, or flesh that is particularly flaccid or drawn, reflect imbalances in this Spleen function.

The Spleen keeps Blood in its vessels. Also as a part of its containment function, the Spleen keeps Blood in its vessels. Bleeding disorders like hemorrhage, frequent bloody nose, and frequent bruising indicate poor function of the Spleen.

The Spleen opens into the mouth and manifests in the lips. As a part of its connection to food, the Spleen opens into the mouth and governs the sense of taste. Although the tongue is governed by the Heart, the sense of taste is related to food and digestion, and therefore to the Earth element.

The lips reflect Spleen function in their color, moistness, and fullness.

The Spleen houses thought. Although the Heart houses the mind, the Spleen governs the quality of thought at the mind's disposal. Clarity of concentration, the ability to do mental work like schoolwork, and memorization are all functions of the Spleen that rely on its ability to center and concentrate.

The Spleen is also called the Spleen-Pancreas. Many modern texts refer to the Spleen as the Spleen-Pancreas, since the Chinese definition of the Spleen includes functions that are attributed to the pancreas in Western medicine—like digestion of foods through enzymes, and the metabolism of sugar.

The Stomach controls the rotting and ripening of food. The most active Yang organ, the Stomach breaks foods down, allowing the Spleen to extract essences.

The Stomach rules descending. The Stomach balances the Spleen's ascending movements by directing the movement of the qi and essences whose proper direction is down. Imbalances of the Stomach's downward direction of qi include nausea, vomiting, and belching.

The meridians that specifically correspond with Earth are the Spleen and Stomach meridians. Together, these meridians distribute the Earth element's energy in the body. The Spleen meridian begins on the big toe and runs along the inner aspect of the leg, along the pubic bone and up the

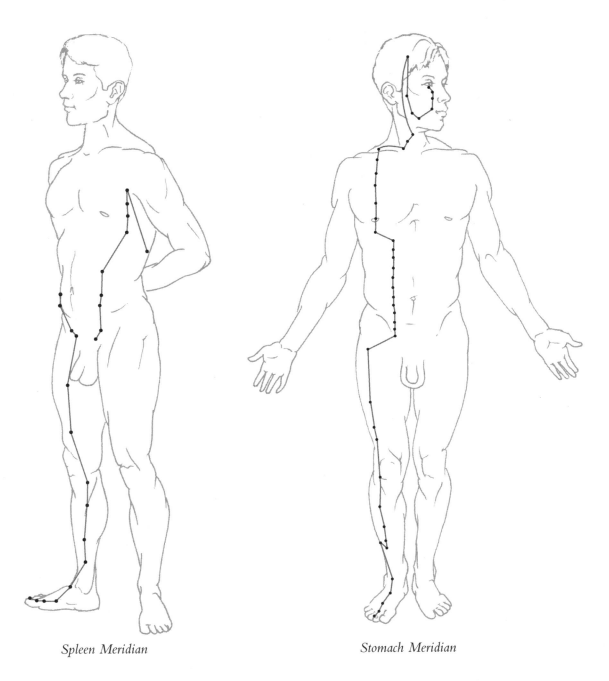

Spleen Meridian

Stomach Meridian

front of the torso before angling off to end on the side of the trunk.

The Stomach meridian begins just below the eye and runs down the front of the face, jaw, neck, and torso, continuing all the way down the outer aspect of the leg to end on the foot at the third toe.

EARTH OUT OF BALANCE

Earth in Deficiency

When Earth is deficient, any or all of its functions may be weak. Therefore an Earth deficiency can manifest in the area of digestion, Blood, thought, or energy. Some common signs of Earth deficiency are:

* fatigue
* loose stools
* pale lips and tongue
* dry skin
* short or scanty menstruation
* hemorrhoids
* poor appetite
* obesity
* mental spaciness
* frequent bruises
* sleepiness after meals

Others include shortness of breath on exertion, dizziness, uterine prolapse, varicose veins, nosebleeds, abdominal noises, gas, feelings of being overwhelmed, poor concentration, diabetes, hypoglycemia, and cravings for sweets. The tongue may have scalloped edges, a thick coat, and/or a swollen body.

Creatively, an Earth deficiency often manifests as someone too tired or too busy to take the time to be creative. They may feel that they lack imagination, talent, or creativity, or they may just lack the energy. In any case, the real or perceived lack signals a deficiency of Earth's generous allowance and nurturing.

Karen R. had a Spleen deficiency that was chronic and clearly marked. Seeking acupuncture for treatment of her fatigue, Karen said she would "crash" after eating, and often had to lie down and sleep for a while immediately after meals. Although this happened mostly when meals were bigger than usual, she would also notice it when she was tired or under stress. Karen had an enormous appetite and craved sweets particularly, even though they caused definite crashes. She was frequently tired during the day, and would develop shakes and sweats if she hadn't eaten in a while. She was frequently dizzy, often cold, often thirsty, and had chronically loose stool. Upon examination, Karen also had several dark bruises on her legs, and confirmed that she bruised very easily.

Karen's condition pointed clearly to Spleen dysfunction, with its signs of fatigue tied to appetite and eating. Her craving for sweets, loose stool, and frequent bruising are also classic Spleen-deficiency signs. With a family history of diabetes and symptoms of a moderate-to-severe nature, Karen was first referred to a physician for blood-sugar testing, though that proved inconclusive. Karen's treatments focused on tonifying her Earth element.

When Earth deficiency is the primary imbalance, the other elements may do the following:

EARTH
deficiency is the primary imbalace

FIRE ↓
may be deficient
and undernourishing
its child

METAL ↑↓
may be deficient because
undernourished, or excess
and draining its mother

WOOD ↑
may be excess and
overcontrolling

WATER ↑
may be excess because
undercontrolled, and may
be "backing up" into Earth

Earth in Excess

Earth excess often develops after prolonged Earth deficiency, when chronic poor digestion creates phlegm that builds up over time to slow and congest body processes. Signs of Earth excess can include:

* muzziness of head
* heavy feeling in head or limbs

*Let us join the
Great Mother,*

*Change blood into
milk, clay into
vessel,*

*egg into child, wind
into song,*

*our bodies into
worship.*

—Elizabeth Roberts

* dull headache
* yeast infection
* sinus congestion
* respiratory phlegm
* lumps and nodules under
  the skin
* obesity
* nausea
* vomiting
* belching
* constipation

Other symptoms include hiccuping, wringing of hands, tendency to worry, tendency to take care of others at expense of oneself, obsessive thoughts, brain "chatter," poor concentration, and muddled thinking. There may also be a thick and sticky coating on the tongue.

Creatively, an excess Earth element just has too much clutter. This may be physical clutter—desks piled high with junk or miscellaneous storage—or mental clutter such as too many unfocused thoughts that fog the mind and render it unable to concentrate.

Richard M. came to acupuncture with a variety of symptoms, the most pressing of which were severe fatigue, a lack of concentration he called "brain fog," and chronic stomach pain, nausea, and belching. Richard also complained of a daily fever, and a thick and cheesy coat on his tongue that got worse when he was tired. His symptoms had come on after a parasitic infestation picked up while traveling abroad, but they had remained for months and months. With overpowering exhaustion and no ability to concentrate, Richard had quit his job and was extremely frustrated by his condition, which no amount of immunological testing had diagnosed.

Richard's is a clear-cut case of Spleen dampness, though other conditions are present as well. The fatigue, cloudy thinking, and Stomach symptoms are all Earth signs, while the nausea, belching, thick tongue coat, and fever point clearly to an excess. Richard's treatments focused on draining dampness, and strengthening his Earth element so that it would create less dampness in the future.

When Earth excess is the primary imbalance, the other elements may realign as follows:

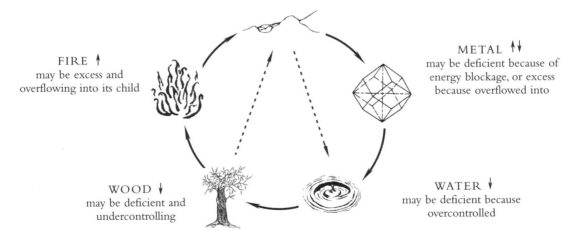

EARTH
excess is the primary imbalace

FIRE ↑
may be excess and
overflowing into its child

METAL ↑↓
may be deficient because of
energy blockage, or excess
because overflowed into

WOOD ↓
may be deficient and
undercontrolling

WATER ↓
may be deficient because
overcontrolled

EARTH AND ACUPUNCTURE

Because the Earth element governs the flesh and the "container" of the body in general, all acupuncture affects these Earth aspects. In a sense, we treat the container so that it may better suit its evolving contents. In addition, acupuncture can be used to treat the Earth element specifically, for which purpose the Five Element points are used.

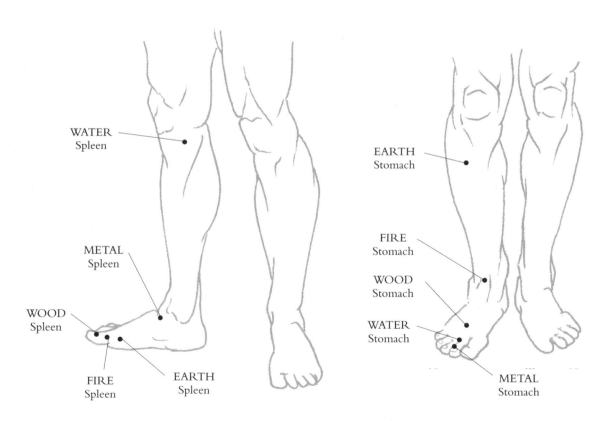

WATER
Spleen

METAL
Spleen

WOOD
Spleen

FIRE
Spleen

EARTH
Spleen

EARTH
Stomach

FIRE
Stomach

WOOD
Stomach

WATER
Stomach

METAL
Stomach

*Five Element Points on
the Spleen Meridian*

*Five Element Points on
the Stomach Meridian*

The **Wood** points on the Earth meridians are used to influence the dynamic between Earth and its controlling element. These Wood points are tonified when Wood needs to control excess Earth, and dispersed when overactive Wood needs to stop overcontrolling Earth.

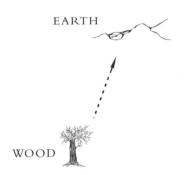

Since Fire is the mother of Earth, the **Fire** points on the Earth meridians are most commonly used to tonify Earth deficiencies through its mother. They can also be dispersed, however, to prevent Fire excess from overflowing into its child.

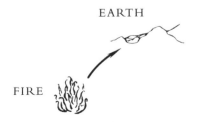

The **Earth** points tonify deficient Earth, and can be used whenever Earth's dynamic needs to be adjusted— to tonify Metal through its mother, for instance, to control Water, or to keep Earth from overcontrolling Water.

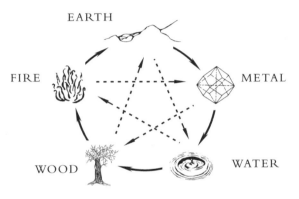

The **Metal** points on the Earth meridians can be tonified to strengthen Metal through its mother, or dispersed to prevent excess Metal from draining its mother.

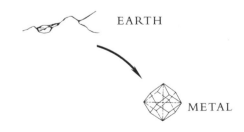

The **Water** points on Earth meridians influence the relationship between Earth and the element it

EARTH

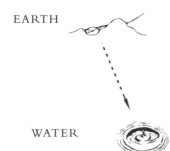

WATER

controls. These points can be dispersed to help Earth control Water excess, or tonified to prevent Earth from overcontrolling Water.

Treatments for Earth Deficiency and Excess

For an Earth deficiency, a common treatment might include Fire points to tonify Earth through its mother, and Wood points to stop Wood from over-controlling Earth.

Karen R.'s treatments for Earth deficiency followed a similar strategy, accomplished through acupuncture needling and dietary modifications. At first Karen had a very hard time cutting down on the sweets in her diet. She also didn't want to eat regular meals (especially breakfast). After a few treatments, however, she felt less tired after meals and had more energy, in general, and these improvements motivated her to make some changes in her habits. Soon Karen began to take better care of herself, nourishing herself with good food and proper sleep, and even actively seeking out people and situations that made her feel good. As Karen's Earth element grew stronger, she was more willing and better equipped to nurture her own needs, which further accelerated her healing process.

For an Earth excess, Wood points would be tonified to control Earth, while Metal points would be dispersed to drain Earth through its child.

Richard's Earth excess was treated with these points, and he improved rapidly. His daily fever stopped after the second treatment, and his brain fog and fatigue cleared up gradually in the succeeding weeks. Richard's stomach pain and nausea took longer to change, in part because he continued to eat many raw and cold foods, which weakened his Earth element.

EARTH AND FOOD

As the primary digestive organs of the body, the Spleen and Stomach have more significant roles in the digestion and metabolism of foods than other organ pairs. Because the proper transformation of foods and fluids is essential to the production of the body's fundamental energy, digestion affects much more than the simple breakdown of foods; it is basically the source of health and illness throughout the body.

Earth school followers, who maintain that Earth "feeds all," found that our health is determined by what we eat and how we eat it. As our only renewable resource besides air and water, food is the fabric out of which we create ourselves every day. If we eat poor quality foods, or are unable to secure good nutrition from them, we have only dirt and refuse from which to power ourselves; on the other hand, if we eat truly healthy foods and can process them effectively, we contribute high-quality goods to the production of our cells, tissues, and processes. Because of this, improper eating habits that weaken the Spleen and Stomach are believed to create disorder and disease in the body. Conversely, eating habits that protect them foster good health.

The Spleen in Chinese medicine is an organ that appreciates moderation and regularity. Like the Earth element of which it is a part, the Spleen represents nurturing care, protection, and balance: Random or careless eating habits disrupt its careful balance, and thereby disturb the integrity of the whole body. Some basic habits that protect the Spleen include eating regular meals (not skipping or eating haphazardly), eating moderately (not overindulging), and eating calmly and with reverence for the food and the Earth from which it came. Eating hurriedly, or when anxious or angry, disrupts bodily processes. Other ways to protect the spleen include the following:

Food should be well chewed. Digestion begins in the mouth, and hurrying through the mouth's processes leaves more work for the rest of the body to do, which often overtaxes it.

Don't eat late at night. The evening meal should be finished at least three hours before going to bed. Otherwise, food still in the body makes demands on resources that should be resting. Eating at night can cause weight gain, indigestion, poor sleep, constipation, and grinding teeth.

Food should be cooked. In general, cold and raw foods damage the Spleen. So the American habit of eating salads and yogurt as "healthy" food is considered quite unhealthy in Chinese medicine. Cold and raw foods create dampness and phlegm, and, ultimately, excess heat, which the body keeps generating to try to warm up and break down the cold and raw.

Beverages should be drunk at room temperature or warmer. The modern habit of drinking liquids straight from the refrigerator, or over ice, is harmful to the Spleen, which cannot tolerate these temperatures. Ideally, water, juice, and other beverages should be drunk at room temperature.

In addition to these general rules, the Spleen is also affected by the energetics of foods, as are the other organs. The Earth element has its corresponding flavor, color, vegetables, and fruits.

Earth's flavor: sweet

The flavor that corresponds to Earth is sweetness. Like other flavors, Earth's flavor has properties of its controlling element, Wood—it tonifies and harmonizes the body's organs and tissues, helping them to "individuate" and strengthen their functions. Sweet foods penetrate the Spleen and Stomach, Earth's corresponding organs, and can therefore direct the healing energies of other foods toward them.

Grains, in general, are considered sweet foods and are therefore highly tonifying, forming the backbone of Taoist cuisine and of most traditional diets. Rice, corn, wheat, barley, rye, amaranth, and quinoa are all staple ingredients, as are potatoes and sweet potatoes. Whatever the choice, these Earth element foods should form fifty to eighty percent of daily dietary intake.

Most meats, fish, beans, and nuts are also considered sweet foods and are highly tonifying, of especial benefit to those with weak constitutions and conditions. Other sweet foods include apples, apricots, cherries, dates, figs, beets, carrots, chard, cucumbers, eggplants, potatoes, shiitake mushrooms, squash, sweet potatoes, almonds, chestnuts, coconuts, sesame seeds, sunflower seeds, and sweeteners. Sweet herbs include licorice, rehmannia, and ginseng.

The sweet flavor used in moderation is good for deficiencies of all kinds. However, eating lots of sweet foods will weaken the Earth element, which may sink into deficiency or stagnate into excess conditions of heat, dampness, and phlegm. Unlike the other flavors, sweetness cannot be eaten to control excesses of its element; it will only aggravate them. Excesses of the sweet flavor can occur when we eat too much of "sweet" foods like meats and fats, or when we eat foods that are themselves too sweet, like refined and concentrated sugars.

These refined sweeteners are too much for the body to handle; they weaken the Spleen, causing dampness and heat in the body. As these foods form a large proportion of most modern diets, many people are afflicted by some form of Spleen imbalance, and would be much better off avoiding refined and concentrated sugars altogether.

Earth's vegetables: layered and tightly packed

Vegetables that align with Earth energies are those that are layered around themselves, like onions, artichokes, and cabbage, or those packed tightly together like corn and wheat. They exemplify Earth's close attention and nurturing, and can be eaten freely during conditions of deficiency or excess.

Earth's fruits: compact

Earth's fruits are dense and tightly packed, like apples and pears. Such density echoes Earth's accumulative nature. Because they are sweet and raw, like all fruits,

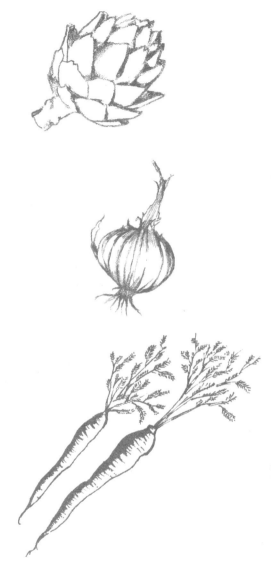

Layered vegetables like artichokes and onions evoke Earth's focused attention, while the orange color of carrots also signals the Earth element.

apples and pears can easily weaken the Spleen, and should be eaten only in moderation in both excess and deficient conditions.

Earth's colors: yellow, orange, and brown

Earth's yellow, orange, and brown foods can be used to tonify Earth deficiencies. Some examples of these foods include corn, carrots, sweet potatoes, yellow squash, pumpkins, brown rice, millet, and barley.

Tonifying Earth Deficiency

The most important factor in an Earth-deficiency diet is to take proper care of the Spleen: This means cooking all foods so that nothing is eaten raw or cold, eating regular meals, and avoiding Spleen-damaging sweeteners and concentrated sugars.

The diet, in general, should be hearty, filling, and balanced. Emphasize yellow Earth-element foods like corn, carrots, sweet potatoes, and squash; round and layered foods like onions, cabbage, artichokes, hazelnuts, and cantaloupe; and plenty of whole grains, including millet, rice, and barley. These foods sustain calmness, feelings of centeredness and balance, and can be included in the diet during any period when these qualities are needed.

In addition, most meats, fish, beans, and nuts are sweet and highly tonifying, and should be liberally included whenever there is deficiency. Meats in particular are extremely grounding, and recommended for people who are spaced out, weak, cold,

Talk of mysteries! Think of our life in nature, daily to be shown matter, to come in contact with it, rocks, trees, wind on our cheeks! The solid earth! The actual world! The common sense! Contact! Contact! Who are we? Where are We?

— Henry David Thoreau, *The Maine Woods*

or otherwise ungrounded. It's also a good idea to include a balance of foods from each of the elements when eating for Earth deficiency; Earth foods should be complemented by foods with each of the other four flavors.

People with Spleen deficiencies often experience cravings for sweets and stimulants, which give a quick rush of energy. Sweets in the form of fruits and natural sugars can be taken in moderation, but cookies, cakes, and refined sugars of all kinds will weaken the Spleen and create more deficiency and more fatigue, as will coffee, chocolate, and tea. It is best simply to follow a more tonifying dietary plan.

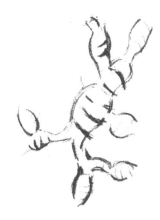

ginger

EARTH-TONIFYING RECIPE
Spicy Gingerbread

½ cup butter

1 egg

2½ cups whole wheat flour

1½ tsp. baking soda

1½ tsp. cinnamon

2 tsps. ginger, grated fresh

½ tsp. salt

¼ tsp. black pepper, finely ground

½ cup blackstrap molasses

½ cup honey

1 cup hot water

1. Melt butter in a large saucepan and let cool slightly. Add egg and beat.
2. In a mixing bowl, combine the dry ingredients.
3. In another bowl, combine blackstrap molasses, honey, and hot water.
4. Pour the contents of the mixing bowls into the saucepan in alternating batches. Mix well and pour into a 9x9-inch greased pan. Bake for 1 hour at 350°F.

Controlling Earth Excess with Food

Unlike other elements, Earth cannot be controlled by increased intake of its flavor, as sweetness is cloying and creates further excess. Grains should be eaten only in small quantities, while fruits and sweeteners should be avoided altogether. Instead, foods from the sour and bitter categories should be emphasized (see Wood and Fire chapters) to control excess Earth. Cooked greens are the most important aspect of a diet to control dampness, and should be eaten frequently. Pungent foods and other Metal-element foods like citrus are helpful for draining dampness, but dairy and soy products will exacerbate it. Alcohol creates a lot of dampness and should not be a part of a dampness-controlling diet.

Diets for Earth excess should be followed whenever there is internal dampness, as well as during humid weather when dampness starts to accumulate in the tissues and bones. As dampness is a slow-moving disorder, it can take a long time to resolve; it requires real changes in eating habits in addition to careful regulation of the kinds of foods eaten. Following the above dietary guidelines for protecting the Spleen is an important start. In addition, the general diet should be light and deliberate.

Meat and fish can be eaten, unless the dampness is also accompanied by Fire signs (infection, throbbing headache, fevers, irritability, yellow tongue coat, red tongue body). With heat, meat consumption should be reduced or avoided completely for one to two weeks, and warming pungents like chilis, black pepper, and onions should be guarded carefully as well.

Candida yeast conditions qualify as dampness in Chinese medicine, and can be partially controlled through a dampness-controlling diet. Most of the candida diets developed by Western practitioners are very similar to Chinese dampness-control diets.

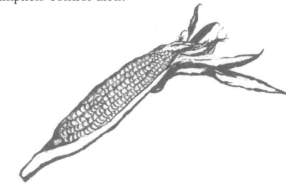

EARTH EXCESS RECIPE
Steamed Corn with Chili-Lime Oil

5 tsp. olive or peanut oil

2 tsp. grated lime zest

$\frac{1}{2}$ tsp. sea salt

$\frac{1}{2}$ tsp. chili powder

2 tbsp. fresh lime juice

5 ears corn

1. Combine the oil, lime zest, sea salt, chili powder, and lime juice in a small bowl.

2. Pull back but don't remove the corn husks, and take out all the corn silk.

3. Brush the corn with the flavored oil and pull husks back on.

4. Add 1 to 2 inches of water to a large pot that has a steamer basket and bring to a boil.

5. Put corn into steamer basket and cover, steaming until corn is tender, 8 to 10 minutes.

EARTH AND QIGONG

The Earth element is vital to the production of two QiGong treasures—Energy and Essence. In addition, Earth's ideals of balance and moderation underlie all QiGong practices, which emphasize appropriate lifestyle as the basis of health, harmony, and longevity. Lifestyle generally includes eating and sleeping habits, rest and work habits, emotional balance and sexual activity. One well-known text, *The Yellow Emperor's Classic of Internal Medicine* (attributed to an emperor who lived in the third millennium B.C.E.), describes the importance of balance as follows:

In the past, people practiced the Tao, the Way of Life. They understood the principle of balance, of yin and yang, as represented by the transformation of the energies of the universe. Thus, they formulated practices such as Dao-in, an exercise combining stretching, massaging, and breathing to promote energy flow, and meditation to help maintain and harmonize themselves with the universe. They ate a balanced diet at regular times, arose and retired at regular hours, avoided overstressing their bodies and minds, and refrained from overindulgence of all kinds. They maintained well-being of body and mind; thus, it is not surprising that they lived over one hundred years. *

The emperor then goes on to describe, in greater detail, how such balances are maintained—by avoiding excessive desire and fantasy, living simply, remaining active without over-working, and so on. Whereas modern Western medicine considers lifestyle factors to be adjuncts to physical factors, the Chinese have always considered lifestyle to be the primary cause and prevention of disease. In their view, an imbalanced life is what renders a body vulnerable to germs, cancers, decay, etc. A balanced lifestyle with balanced behaviors, on the other hand, will be able to counter any undue influence before it becomes a serious disease.

A balanced lifestyle from a Taoist point of view includes the following:

Regularity. Routine is the modus operandi of the Earth element. Like the clockwork timing of sunrise and sunset, and the regular turning of the seasons, Earth thrives on a routine schedule of regular waking and sleeping times, regular mealtimes, and regular work hours. Disruptions in these routines destabilize Earth, and set the stage for further, more extreme imbalances.

Sufficient amounts of work and rest. Balancing work and rest is important to the stability of the overall being. Many people don't know how to relax fully, and don't allow themselves enough time for sleep and play; they become stressed out, and unable to properly accommodate the needs of their

* From *The Yellow Emperor's Classic of Internal Medicine.*

bodies. Eventually, they exhaust the body's supplies of Energy and Essence. On the other hand, too little activity—a sedentary lifestyle—can lead to stagnation. Good health can be maintained only by engaging in activity and rest at appropriate times.

Balanced mental and emotional habits. Balancing the mind and the emotions is a concept not well understood in the West, but it requires discipline and wisdom. The idea is to refrain from thinking too hard, worrying too much, or indulging excessively in any emotion. By maintaining a certain detachment, we protect our minds and bodies from the weaknesses that would make them vulnerable to disease.

Avoiding overindulgence. Overindulgence has specific referents in QiGong and Chinese medical practice, and most commonly refers to excessive sex, which squanders Kidney essence. Overeating and excessive luxury are also considered overindulgences. Like excessive emotion, indulgent behaviors overbalance us and create weakness.

Besides attaining longevity, QiGong

masters are sometimes able to accomplish things considered impossible in a modern scientific age. Great healers, they are also capable of incredible feats of strength and endurance as well as psychic and psychokinetic activity. Such "supernatural" capacities have long been attributed to masters of QiGong and Yoga, who credit balance and discipline for their accomplishments.

EARTH AND FENG SHUI

The Earth element is as central to our external environment as it is to our individual bodies. Evident in our homes and offices and in the very formations of the planet itself—mountains, rocks, hills, soil, and clay, Earth also manifests in the colors yellow and brown, and in every kind of container that we surround ourselves with. Earth not only feeds all; in the realm of Feng Shui it holds all as well.

Outdoors, soil is an important indicator of the overall health of a site. In Feng Shui as in agriculture, soil is evaluated on the basis of its richness and fertility. Moist, loamy, and living soils are conducive to life and health; they indicate abundant and free-flowing qi, and therefore imply a good location for home or business. Dry and barren soils, on the other hand, or overly rocky ones, reveal a weak Earth element and are unpropitious signs for the placement of a home or business.

Hills and mountains, in general, are Earth element formations, and are considered vital to a site by classical Feng Shui practitioners. In fact, Earth "dragons"—strong Earth formations like rolling hills—are one of the two main factors in determining the ideal spot for a house on a site.

Ideal hills are rolling and not too steep or craggy. Houses should be nestled within the hills, preferably facing them. However, if mountains slope too steeply, their qi is considered unstable and dangerous; too close to a house, mountain qi is overbearing. A shield of bamboo or other trees would be necessary to screen a dwelling from these perilous influences.

In more urban environments, buildings take the place of mountains in representing the Earth element. Unusually tall or close buildings can be overbearing like a too-steep mountain, and should be deflected so they don't damage the qi of the people living near-by. A mirror hung facing the offending building will reflect its qi back to it, so it no longer oppresses neighbors. Alternatively, a small mirror or a pool of water on the roof of the smaller building will have the same effect.

The shape that more specifically corresponds to the Earth element is an elevated but flattened expanse. Mountains with flat mesas or plateaus, and buildings that are more horizontal than vertical are particularly associated with Earth. Bridges, which form flat plateaus over gaps and waters, also represent Earth.

Indoors, Earth shapes are flat across the top like plateaus: tables, desks, shelves, beds, sofas, and chairs all represent the Earth element in a home or office. In addition, anything that holds or contains anything else has a strong Earth component—vases, bowls, bottles, as well as bureaus and closets. Cross beams are also considered Earth, as they create an Earth shape by joining two upright beams.

Earth *colors* are yellow, brown, and beige, as well as tones like adobe and

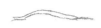 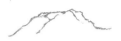 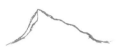 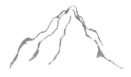

brick. These colors are especially appropriate in living rooms and dens—the centers of family life. Earth *materials* are anything made of clay or brick—pottery, dishware, potting soil.

Rolling hills, like the first three shown above, are ideal sites for homes, businesses, and ancestral graves. Steeper peaks, like the fourth illustration, are unstable and therefore unpropitious sites for building.

Tonifying Earth Deficiency

Adding Earth to tonify a deficiency can be as simple as bringing home a new teapot or vase. Containers and vessels, particularly in clay, add security and homeyness to any environment. Bottles and jars—new canisters for food or tools—will support a weak and undernourished Earth element, while larger Earth containers like chairs and bureaus are perfect for stabilizing an ungrounded Earth.

Add yellows and browns to your visual field in the form of clothing, decorative items, jewelry, craft projects, and so on. Wear yellows and browns to help you focus thought into words when you have speaking, writing, or studying to do. Let some sunflowers or black-eyed Susans ground and center your inner confusions.

A good way to heighten a weak Earth element is just to be aware of the nurturing and containing capabilities of the soft chairs, sofas, serving bowls, and decorative baskets that are present in every household. Practice being enfolded in beds and chairs, and practice enfolding daily objects in secure and generous spaces. Serve the foods and beverages you eat in attractive bowls and cups, arrange flowers lovingly in a vase, hang clothes safely in the closet. Notice the care that containment implies, and bestow it upon yourself; Earth element's most common complaints stem from being ignored.

In addition, try tonifying Fire, as described in the Fire chapter, to strengthen Earth through its mother.

The quickest way to control an excess Earth element is to clean up clutter. Not dirt necessarily, which is the province of the Metal element, but the clutter and overabundance that accumulate around us during times of stress and inattention. Clean off tabletops and desktops, clean out drawers and cabinets, organize closets and basements, throwing out as much as you can, and organizing the rest into neat piles. This will begin the process of draining and simplifying an overburdened Earth element.

Secondarily, follow the instructions in the Wood chapter for tonifying Wood, which will then control Earth.

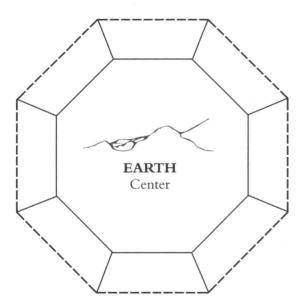

EARTH
Center

The Ba-Gua area that corresponds to Earth is the center; it can be used to tonify deficiency or control excess.

Place a small round or hexagonal carpet in the center of a room to strengthen the Earth element there, or place a table or coffee table in the center area. Alternatively, you can hang a mobile or a wind chime from the center of the ceiling. If there is a light fixture in the center of the ceiling, make sure it is clean and supplied with fresh, bright bulbs. Try painting or replacing the fixture with one that is yellow or red.

A healthy Earth element establishes a stable foundation for the energy and activity of our lives. The foods we eat, the

Nature was my first mother.
I memorized the forest floor as I would
my mother's body. This forest skin
smelled like pine sap and sweet rot, and
it stained my diapers green and
perfumed my hair, which was always
tangled with bits of leaves, small sticks,
and moss. It never occurred to me
during those early years in the forest
that I was human.

—Brenda Peterson, *Nature and Other Mothers*

homes we live in, the money we spend, and the people we connect with all rely on the powerfully nourishing forces of the Earth element. Because it governs the real nuts and bolts of survival, like eating and spending, Earth brings a level of practicality to our endeavors that would otherwise be lacking. It teaches us that a certain amount of living is repetitive work—"We all gotta do what we all gotta do," and there's no getting around it. But once we understand this basic truth, and can engage in the routine work with dedication and with joy, a whole new dimension of being emerges. We slowly learn that life's most golden moments are achieved through such work, not in spite of it. The happiness we seek comes from channeling everything—our sweat, our tears, our joys, and our inspirations—to the journey of growth. These realizations bring Earth's nourishing into Metal's wisdom, where we discover what the journey is about.

CHAPTER 5

METAL

GOLD, JEWELS, AND CRYSTALS EVOKE THE SYMBOLOGY of Metal in myths and fairy tales around the world. A prize of immeasurable value, treasure is the reason for every quest and the goal of every hero. The Holy Grail, the dragon's treasure, and the philosopher's gold are all versions of the same tale: the search for something uncorrupted. Often this treasure takes the form of a special princess or prince, whose beauty or innocence identifies them with uncorrupted purity.

The treasure in these stories is generally protected by conditions that make it dangerous to seek and difficult to obtain: Perilous journeys, diabolical creatures, magic spells, and evil magicians safeguard the treasure from all hands. Only the most valiant and honorable seekers ever gain the treasure, and even they are sorely tested along the journey, having to prove themselves worthy again and again. When the hero and heroine succeed and live happily ever after, they are eternally enriched by the gold they have achieved.

In accordance with Carl Jung's pioneering work with myth and dream, the treasures in these myths can be understood as symbols of self-knowledge, and the questing journeys as humanity's search for the same. The jewels are thus pearls of wisdom, won by dint of hard work, honesty, and pure intention. The alchemist's fabled quest to turn lead into gold is likewise a pursuit of internal enlightenment. Metal in these stories thus represents wisdom and self-knowledge—the true riches of life.

Weaponry is another aspect of Metal that appears in myths and fairy tales. Swords, spears, and knives represent a symbolic scything—a separation of forces like pure from impure, or good from evil. When weapons are used, it is a sign of elimination: Some part is being discarded for the health of the whole. Whether an evil giant has been killed or a valiant hero wounded, the weapon acts as an agent of change, removing something no longer necessary to the kingdom or the man.

Metal in the Five Element cycle signals both the process of refinement and the pure essence that is its product: the Holy Grail as well as the search for it. It signifies loss and reduction, but also an indestructible purity that remains when all else is gone. Metal's learning and discerning, its questing and heroics, are archetypally masculine attributes, just as Earth's nurturing is quintessentially feminine. The Metal element thus represents archetypal father energy, which compels the masculine part of each of us to journey forth to seek treasure, to slay dragons, and to teach our hard-won wisdom to those who walk the road behind us.

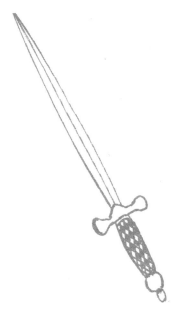

Swords and other weapons embody Metal's attributes of separation and elimination.

EARTH

FIRE

METAL

WOOD

WATER

In the Creation cycle, Metal is the child of Earth. Whereas growth is nurtured unconditionally in the Earth phase, in Metal it is more actively directed; unproductive or used resources are dispensed with while valuable products are retained and refined. In the Control cycle, Metal is controlled by Fire, which melts it. Metal's qualities of discernment and separation can be obliterated by Fire's melting and merging of distinctions.

In the natural world, metal is formed deep inside the earth, where high temperatures and pressures cause molecules in molten magma to separate into homogeneous layers. Some layers cool quickly into volcanic basalts, while others condense gradually into minerals and ores. Still others stack themselves in precise latticelike structures to form crystals. This process of separation pushes away impurities and molecules of dissimilar composition, forming metals that are pure and distinct.

In the Five Element cycle, Metal characterizes a similar process of separation. Formed in the nurturing energies of the Earth phase, Metal separates that which is spent, impure, or unnecessary from that which is pure. While impure waste is eliminated, pure essences are further refined, valued as treasure or sometimes stored for later use. This process of elimination can be difficult, but Metal is an exceptionally strong element precisely because of it: Elimination strips away impurities to concentrate essence. The Metal element is naturally aligned with the mineral kingdom, and shares its hardness as well as its shine.

In the YinYang cycle, Metal signifies the ascendance of Yin. Following the Yang expansiveness of Wood and Fire, and Earth's mediated transition, the Metal phase begins to manifest Yin's inward movement: Objects show signs of introversion, contraction, and quieting. On a physical level, Metal refines the energies that were nurtured in the Earth phase and converts them into potential that is stored for later use. The storage function of Metal is the successor of Earth's containment—whereas Earth does the containing, Metal represents what is contained.

Metal corresponds to autumn in the cycle of the seasons. In autumn, the sap that is the life-force of every plant withdraws from its leaves and branches to collect in the roots. Nutrients stored underground in this way retain their potency through long, cold winters. At the same time, the tree's vessels channel impurities upward into the leaves, where they will be discarded with the fall. Though beautiful in their time, leaves cease to be functional in winter's relative darkness, so the trees stop nourishing them and they fall away.

Autumn's cool temperatures and shortened daylight hours signal the growing dominance of Yin. Animals and plants become more Yin as well, turning inward to build up the stores of nutrients they'll need to get them through the long winter. Whereas trees store nutrients as sap, animals store them as fat, converting everything they eat (which is a lot, in fall!) into fat, which is the densest form of energy storage. Fat protects animals from cold, and can be converted into energy when food supplies are scarce.

Autumn is also a harvest time, when markets are piled high with red and gold apples, late corn, wheat and oats, broccoli, potatoes, and so on. The crops we reap have condensed their bounty into nutritious fruit and vegetable organs; our harvesting of them is a process of retaining their essence while discarding the husks and stalks that are no longer necessary. Traditionally, autumn has also been a time of canning and drying, slaughtering and salting, as we store up the resources vital to our survival in scarcer winter months.

In the cycle of a day, Metal governs late afternoon and evening—when day draws to a close. Yang daylight gives way to Yin darkness while people return to their homes, relax, and engage in relatively passive activities like eating and talking. Evening is often family time, when extraneous friends and relatives are pared away and the immediate family collects—like a refined essence—to spend its time together. In general, Metal hours involve winding down, letting go the cares of the day, and preparing for the night's rest.

In the construction of a building, Metal is the period of completion, when workers put on the

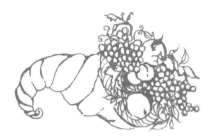

At harvest time,
we reap the benefits of
what we have sown,
engaging Metal's
energies of distillation
and preservation.

finishing touches, make final adjustments, and cart away the garbage and materials that are no longer necessary. As a building reaches completion, it no longer needs the input and industry it once did—it is functional on its own and may already be housing its occupants and/or businesses, though the final work is still being done. The removal of garbage is an important part of this process, as the true essence of the building can be revealed only when the waste has been eliminated.

In any creative endeavor Metal likewise governs the finishing phase, when we put our efforts into refining our project and perfecting the details that express its essence. At this stage we stain wood to bring out the beauty of its grain, plate and garnish a dish, or retool a sentence until it reads just right. At the same time, we remove superfluity and waste until what remains is a completed, perfect thing.

Cleansing processes also owe their strength to Metal energies. In cleaning, we consolidate the essence of something by removing impurities from it. Whether it's hair, a countertop, or a backyard, cleaning makes things "shine" by disemburdening them of the elements that don't belong to them, thus revealing their essence. Metal's cleansing is a physical removal of dirt, as opposed to Earth's straightening, which establishes order out of chaos.

The mental correlate of cleaning is Metal's separation and judgment. The process of discerning urgent from not urgent, present from past, or essence from surplus calls upon Metal's attribute of separating the pure from the impure. Like the weapons in fairy-tale adventures, discerning kills off what is no longer useful for our immediate purposes.

Although the Fire element's Small Intestine rules discerning, its separative functions are different than those of the Metal element. The Small Intestine separates subjective truth from untruth—discerning the nature of our innermost feelings. Metal, on the other hand, distinguishes on a more external level, separating into categories what is here or not here, crucial or not crucial, and so on. Metal divides and organizes our daily experience.

Judgment uses Metal's sword to eliminate confusion and chaos; it can be a noble process or a destructive one, depending on how thoughtfully it

The Dry Season

*The grasses are tall
and tinted*

*Straw-gold hues of
dryness,*

*and the contradicting
awryness*

*of the dusty roads
a-scatter*

*with pools of colorful
leaves,*

*with the ghosts of the
dreaming year.*

—Kwesi Brew

is employed. In a Solomonic sense, judgment calls upon our higher powers to discern the best action in a given circumstance. It can help us adjudge the value of a couch we're about to sell, or the proper way to conduct ourselves at the office picnic; appropriate judgment guides our behavior and gives us a sense of what is right. In its purest form judgment is a recognition of "higher" truth—whether spiritual or social—that transcends individual pettiness and is delivered without negative intent. Legal systems institutionalize this ideal, hoping to preserve "justice" with their codes and practices.

When Metal is distorted, however, judgment can be cruel, often devolving into a tool for punishment. People with an imbalance in this aspect of Metal may be self-righteous and overly judgmental of others, or they may turn the angry sword of judgment upon themselves. Overbearing judgment leads to sadistic and punishing behavior, which finds people focusing on penalties and retribution instead of on the necessity of upholding right action.

Cosmologically, Metal would correspond to a shrinking and condensing of the universe, which has been hypothesized as a future occurrence but never verified. Some physicists expect that the universe will not expand continuously, but will at some point begin to shrink backward toward a denser state, in a mirror-image process of the Big Bang. This would be in keeping with the Five Element theory, which establishes condensation and shrinking as an ineluctable phase of any growth process.

The Metal phase of the menstrual cycle occurs around days twenty-one to twenty-eight. At this time, cells in the ovary begin to degenerate (provided fertilization has not occurred), and they cease to produce the hormones that help blood vessels supply the lining of the uterus. Without a proper blood supply, the uterine cells die off, to be shed when menstruation begins. Like the dying and falling of autumn leaves, the degeneration and dying of cells is emblematic of the Metal phase, in which living systems are on the decline.

The forces of Autumn create dryness in Heaven and metal on Earth; they create the lung organ and the skin upon the body . . . and the nose, and the white color, and the pungent flavor . . . the emotion grief, and the ability to make a weeping sound.

—The Yellow Emperor's Classic of Internal Medicine

Metal on a climatic scale manifests as dryness. Like Metal, dryness represents a process of reduction and contraction. It's a somewhat paradoxical concept that implies both the process of draining and the consolidated materials left behind when a field or container has been drained.

Drying in nature is the logical successor of dampness. After humid summer, autumn drains moisture, including its important nutrients, away from leaves and branches into roots. The leaves become dry and fall off, but the roots store through the cold winter the moist essences that will be needed for new growth in the spring. The dryness and death of the leaves are integral parts of this cycle of regrowth—it is only by releasing their leaves that trees can collect the sap they need at their roots.

Similarly, after rains wash away impurities from plants and soils, they leave behind soil that is richer in minerals and nutrients. Repeated runoff and consolidation contribute to the formation of fertile land—like the Nile valley, made richer every year by the deposits of silt left on its banks as the floodwaters of the river recede.

Dryness indicates that something has been lost or removed. Dry weather astringes damp air and soil and prevents or tempers rot, while dryness in the body—in the form of the Metal element—filters breath through the lungs and food mass through the bowels to isolate their essence and eliminate impurities.

But too much dryness leads to parching and paucity. The removal of too much may not leave enough behind, like parched earth that cracks and cannot nourish a seed. Strip-mining leaves the earth naked and nonarable because it removes all the essence in its single-minded pursuit of ore. Clear-cutting, overgrazing, and overfarming, likewise, leave barren lands behind them.

In the body, too much drying renders us as cracked and vulnerable as a droughty plain. Most noticeably, skin grows stiff and flaky, chapping and cracking, especially on the face and hands. Dry coughs are also common, and dry hair, as well as constipation resulting from a lack of fluids in the bowels. Dryness indicates an absence of vital fluids—the essence has been removed along with the impurities.

Environmentally, dryness is spareness, paucity, starkness. Whether it feels like purity or poverty, the absence of anything extra typifies the Metal phase. Arid lands, ascetic monks, fasting diets, and stark interiors all display Metal's sharp edge; minimalism is a Metal value.

Emotionally, Metal is classically associated with grief—the act of letting go, and the process of mourning our losses. Because it hurts us so badly, most people try to avoid grief; they don't want to experience its pain. Others associate grief with weakness, and don't want to give in to debility. It is therefore common practice to ignore grief, denying its very existence in all but the most extreme circumstances. Each new painful situation threatens our bulwark of denial, however, and we become more and more rigid about controlling our feelings. We deny ourselves the right to feel even small things for fear of triggering something we won't be able to control.

Unfortunately, the continued habit of pushing grief away does not really abolish it; it only creates a monster inside us that drains our energy and dampens all our emotions. For when we anesthetize ourselves against pain, we also lose the ability to feel other things, like creativity, love, and joy in full measure. We become numb and dissociated from our own experience.

Grief has its place like all emotions, however, and it must be honored if we are to remain in contact with ourselves. In fact, when we do find the courage to admit grief into our lives, we find that it creates strength instead of weakness. Grief allows us to confront our losses and move through them, letting go of ideas, behaviors, and relationships that are no longer available.

Although the process of mourning our losses is acutely painful, it ultimately brings many gifts, crystallizing what is most important to us. In all its enormity, grief reminds us of how much love we can feel, and there is no greater strength than this deeply humanizing experience. Grief also teaches us what we value in our lives and in the lives of others, giving us the opportunity to redirect our energies toward becoming who we most want to be.

Truly honoring grief involves mourning every loss we feel, even those we don't believe we "ought to" feel, like small ones, or ones that are due to transitions we ourselves initiated. Thus, we grieve inside for favorite possessions we've lost, but also for our old house even when we're moving to a bigger, nicer one. We may grieve over a job we have quit, or for our singleness on the verge of a marriage with someone we love. Grief is not about regret, it is about release.

Resolve is the gift that comes after grief: It is the recognition of what we still have and the decision to move forward with it. It is not hope, exactly, or even determination, just a surprising realization that something of great value remains with us despite or even because of our loss. "What doesn't kill me makes me stronger" is one way of describing it, though this expression excludes the awe and wonder that are the gift of raw suffering.

Resolve emerges from grief like pure gold emerging from ashes; it is the distilled essence of what we had—a person, a love, a home, an experience— and becomes a part of us that we can never lose. Implanted in our hearts, our bones, and our memories, these experiences weave themselves into the fabric of our being and make us more than we were. Resolve hardens in us and pushes us forward into life, where we miraculously discover the ability to feel good again. We love the new house, enter the new marriage with enthusiasm, and feel joy again after losing someone we love not as a salve to our diminished selves, but as deeper, fuller, and richer beings, all the more so for having been tempered by our losses. These are Metal's precious attributes, which make us richer for our experience.

METAL IN THE HUMAN LIFE CYCLE

In the human life cycle, Metal stretches from late-middle into old age. At this stage, people become more Yin than Yang—turning inward rather than pushing outward as they had done in their youths. They become stiffer and slower, less supple than they were in bygone days, and they also become more rigid emotionally—more fixed in their attitudes and less responsive to persuasion. Such fixity is characteristic of the Metal element and a marked contrast to Wood's flexible and adaptive behaviors.

Also at this time, body functions begin to deteriorate, reflecting Metal's qualities of release. With the weakening of hearing, eyesight, memory, or other senses, elders tend to turn inward mentally as well, becoming more absorbed in internal experiences than in the outer world. They grow more reflective, and spend more time reminiscing,

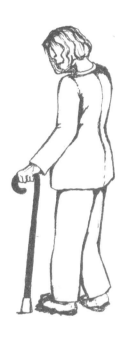

In the Metal phase of our lives we begin to turn inward—physically, mentally, and emotionally.

remembering childhood experiences, and summing up their successes and failures. These behaviors distill the experiences of life into wisdom, which collects like sap in the hearts and minds of aging adults. The image of the old sage, though not highly visible in Western culture, perfectly typifies the condensation during the Metal phase of what's truly valuable in an organism.

At this stage, many older adults also find themselves paring down their environments—moving to smaller homes, selling off or giving away belongings, and reducing the circles of their friends and activities. These typically Metal behaviors mark a refinement and a reduction of Earth's accumulative capacity.

Tara R., now in her early sixties, often talks with her friends about the urge they share to give away a lot of the "stuff" they acquired in their middle years. The antiques they used to collect, the jewelry, and the silver that's been passed on for generations are all slowly moving to their children's houses, church sales, and other recipients. Though their children are sometimes uncomfortable with this behavior (because it looks like a

preparation for death), Tara and her friends feel that it's just natural to be disemburdening themselves of extra objects at this time.

On a spiritual level, Metal exemplifies innocence. Not innocence in a legal sense, but the kind of purity that precludes judgment, allowing all living creatures the right to exist and pursue their dreams without fear of punishment. When we are truly innocent, there is always time to become our best selves, always another chance, always more opportunity to fulfill destiny. No matter how old, how tired, or how disappointed we are, redemptive innocence is available to remind us we are never past healing and never beyond hope. Metal's pure spirit knows we are always eligible for grace.

Many people are wounded in this aspect of spirit, feeling unworthy or tainted as a result of childhood trauma, religious guilt, or social conditioning. They may seek psychological counseling, religion, or a personal spiritual path in an effort to recover their sense of purity. Such institutions provide many ways of becoming innocent again, maintaining rituals that help people peel away the layers of their dis-ease (be it

*My spirit is tuned
to the spring
season:*

*At the fall of
the year there
is autumn in
my heart.*

*Thus imitating
cosmic changes*

*My cottage becomes
a universe.*

—Lu Yun

sin, faithlessness, or ignorance) and find redemption.

Some achieve this purity through rituals of penance like confession, while others purify through the discipline of an austere lifestyle, diet, or meditative practice. Still others achieve purity through the fires of incense and candlelight, through ritual bathing and baptism, or simply through prayer. Whether someone is "born again" or engaged in the process of "healing their inner child," they are cleansing themselves of some perceived impurity so that their remaining essence becomes pure again.

The soul of Metal is wisdom, the treasure hidden at the base of every hardship. Wisdom turns experience into understanding, allowing us to know more about the present because of what we have learned from the past. When we are wise we see more nuances in every situation. We understand dynamics, and can make better, more informed decisions about our actions. Like a well-made sword, wisdom is a tool that allows us to cut through nonsense and see a situation as it really is.

The soul is a strict master, however, teaching us life's lessons through the agency of grief and loss. It requires that we extract our growth from pain, turning disappointment, hurt, and anger into mirrors of self-discovery. This is a difficult path that some people cannot follow; those who can't let go of their hurts will never see them transformed into gifts. People who insist upon learning from their difficulties, however, grow stronger and wiser with each passing day. Every experience adds further distinction to their countenance.

The soul of Metal also creates teachers; those who pass their wisdom on to others. The gift of teaching is a positive aspect of loss—we are none the poorer for giving our wisdom away, provided it is properly valued by those who receive it. Though we are burnt and hammered in the struggles of life, Metal's diligence transforms our shapelessness into a strong and balanced tool, which others can use to navigate life more easily.

Metal in a relationship presides over all separations, whether caused by betrayal, death, or a natural parting of the ways. While Fire and Earth describe the pull toward and connection with others, we also have a strong desire to separate from others.* There can be no outreach without a corresponding in-reach, just as there can be no Yang without Yin: Individuals in a relationship must have adequate time, space, and ability to develop those aspects of themselves that are unique and not dependent on any external relationship.

The Metal element's qualities of purification and letting go play an important role in the separative aspect of a healthy relationship: In the Metal phase we break the energetic bonds created in Earth. While it's a necessary stage of development, it is undeniably painful as we tear away the threads that connect us to those we have loved.

The Metal phase occurs in relationships when friendships or romances break up, or when someone dies. Whether there has been an active schism or a slow attrition, the break-down and reorganization of the Metal phase begins when separation becomes a fact. It requires that we redraw our boundaries to exclude those from whom we're separating—we experience loss, grief, and real disorientation as we struggle to redefine our intimate circle.

The Metal phase also occurs with a child's coming of age. Although a young adult exists within the Fire phase of her own life cycle, her relationship with her parents goes through a Metal phase as she separates her life from theirs and learns to rely on her own strengths for her basic life needs. Traditionally, this phase has been marked by some sort of coming-of-age

* Thomas Moore examines these opposing pulls in his book *SoulMates*.

ceremony, which initiates adolescents into adulthood by virtue of physical, mental, emotional, and/or spiritual trials. These initiations empower the Metal element by acknowledging the transition; they dramatize the loss of childhood as well as the pain and fear involved in separation from its comforts.

In modern life, however, the drama of the transition from childhood to adulthood has been all but lost. We have no vocabulary for acknowledging the pain of separation from our parents, the grief of losing their security and comfort, or the fear of having to survive in an adult world. We call it "adolescence" but we do not recognize that grief will naturally accompany it, as both children and parents experience the breaking of Earth's bonds of interdependence. Partly because of the unacknowledged grief of adolescence, many modern adults go through psychological upheavals later in life, first experiencing the pains of betrayal and separation from their parents in psychotherapy sessions in their twenties and thirties, or even later. Because we have lost our understanding of the emotional nuances of adolescence, additional years and strategies are now required in order to bring about maturity.

In every relationship, the Metal phase manifests as disagreement. Not the posturing and maneuvering of power struggles, but the honest disagreements that occur, prompting both parties to realize that they are, indeed, separate people. It can cause terrible pain if one person in a partnership wants to live in a city, for instance, while the other craves the stillness of the country, or when one loves a person that the other dislikes. Compromises and resolutions do take place, of course, but the pain of the difference remains.

These pains may find us withdrawing into grief, moodiness, quietude, or depression, emotions that pull us back from our constant outpourings of attention and affection. In these darker Metal moods we're invited to commune with our inner selves and our gods, so beginning the transition from Metal to Water.

METAL IN THE BODY

In the body, Metal manifests as the organs and meridians of the Lung (Yin) and the Large Intestine (Yang). These organs govern Metal's functions of release, resolve, purification, and grief, in addition to the following physiological attributes.

The Lungs refine and regulate qi. The Lungs use Metal's powers of refinement to purify the Heavenly qi that they draw into the body during inhalation. Extracting the purest essences from the air they draw in, the Lungs distribute these pure essences to the body while eliminating impurities through exhalation.

Impaired function of this aspect of the Lungs can result in fatigue or other signs of deficient qi, or in breathing difficulties like asthma.

The Lungs defend the body from invasion by colds and flus. Metal's weaponry in the body forms the first line of defense against illness: The Lungs distribute a particular kind of protective qi to the surface of the body, where it keeps germs from invading. As a part of this defensive system, the Lungs control the opening and closing of the pores. They also regulate sweat, which can force sickness out of the body. Dysfunctions in this aspect of the Lungs results in colds and flu, or in sweating disorders.

The Lungs dry the body by dispersing fluids. The Lungs act out Metal's drying function by dispersing body fluids toward points of elimination, like sweat to the skin and urine to the Bladder. When weak Lungs fail to disperse body fluids, dampness can accumulate, causing mucus and phlegm.

The Lungs manifest in the skin and body hair. As a function of their control over body defenses, the Lungs rule the surface of the body and the tissues present there. The Lungs' energy can thus be evaluated in the quality of the skin and body hair, be they moist or dry, limp or elastic, shining or dull, rough or soft.

The Lungs open into the nose. The Lungs govern the sense of smell and the clarity of the nasal passages. The sense of smell is a physical expression of Metal's ability to form judgments: Our noses tell us what is fresh or rotten, attractive or unattractive, and thus helps us to make distinctions and choices. When we "follow our noses" we learn to follow our instinctive judgments.

The Large Intestine rules elimination. A physical counterpart of Metal's loss, the Large Intestine rules the elimination of wastes and impure essences from the body in the form of feces. Dysfunctions in the Large Intestine's energy can result in constipation, diarrhea, or an inability to "let go" of situations or attitudes.

A portion of Metal's energy also manifests in the meridians of the Lung and the Large Intestine. The Lung meridian begins at the edge of the chest and runs down the inner aspect of the arm and palm to end on the thumb.

The Large Intestine meridian begins at the tip of the forefinger and runs up the edge of the forearm to the back of the arm. It goes along the shoulder and the side of the neck, passing through the cheek and crossing beneath the nose to end beside the opposite nostril.

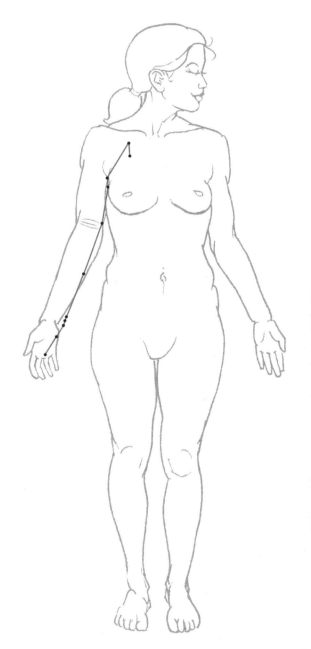

Lung Meridian

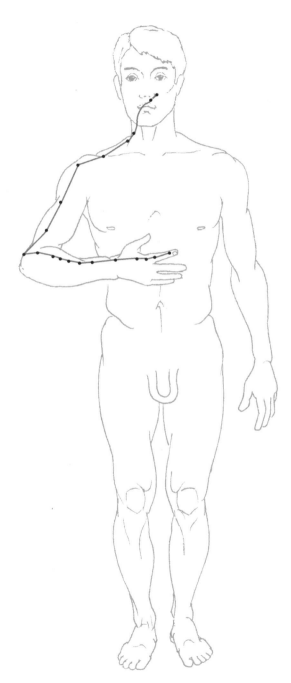

Large Intestine Meridian

METAL OUT OF BALANCE

As is true for all the elements, a Metal imbalance can begin in the body, the mind, the emotions, or the external environment. Wherever it begins, however, an imbalance is likely to cause physical symptoms over time, and the body will manifest signs of Metal deficiency or Metal excess.

Metal in Deficiency

When Metal is deficient, it fails to perform its refining and letting-go processes effectively. Some of the most common Metal-deficiency signs are:

* ★ shortness of breath on exertion
* ★ generally dry skin or body hair
* ★ fatigue
* ★ cold or flu
* ★ too much or not enough sweating
* ★ weak cough or asthma
* ★ overly bright or shiny complexion
* ★ a weak voice
* ★ constipation
* ★ exhaustion
* ★ inability to grieve
* ★ repeating the same destructive patterns of behavior over and over again

Creatively, people with Metal deficiency have difficulty completing their projects. Such people often label themselves perfectionists, because they usually find that their project needs a few more things here, a jot there, etc., but the truth is they just can't let go. Perfectionism masks fears of the loss and separation that accompany completion, and also indicates fears of being harshly judged—all of which are clear signs of Metal imbalance.

When Metal is deficient, the other elements may be pulled out of balance as well. The most likely patterns of imbalance are shown below.

Patrick R. suffered from asthma accompanied by a cough, along with copious respiratory mucus that was frothy and white. Patrick also reported frequent dizziness, persistent fatigue, and chronic sinus congestion. He would sweat easily and abundantly, and mentioned that this had been the case since childhood. Patrick also had a pale but bright complexion and a slightly tremulous voice when tired. When he first came for acupuncture, Patrick also mentioned a book he had been trying to write for four years, but which he was having trouble finishing.

Patrick has a variety of asthma known as "stomach asthma" in Chinese medicine.

EARTH ↓
Metal's mother may
be deficient, and failing
to nourish its child

FIRE ↑
the control element,
may by excess
and overcontrolling

When METAL
deficiency is primary

WOOD ↑
normally controlled by
Metal, may be excess
because undercontrolled

WATER ↑↓
Metal's child may be
deficient if it is
undernourished by its
mother, or may be excess
and draining its mother

In Five Element terms, this is a Metal deficiency exacerbated by a weak Earth element failing to nourish it. Patrick's Metal deficiency is readily apparent in the asthma, cough, and frequent sweating, as well as the distinctive pale-bright complexion and weak voice that are characteristic of Lung dysfunction. Earth deficiency compounds the problem by failing to transform fluids properly, creating mucus in the Lungs and sinuses, which further impairs them. Patrick's fatigue is a result of combined Earth and Metal deficiency, which fails to produce enough qi to give him energy.

Metal in Excess

When Metal is excess, it performs its functions of elimination and purification too severely, or with more energy than is warranted, resulting in a buildup of heat. Some common signs of Metal excess include:

* dry skin or mucus membranes
* profuse nasal or respiratory mucus which may be yellow or green
* swollen tonsils
* deep and phlegmy cough
* dry constipation or crampy diarrhea
* stuffiness in the chest or head
* skin breakouts like rashes, hives, acne, eczema, or psoriasis
* pain or inflammation along the Lung or Large Intestine channels
* neurotic behavior
* being overly judgmental of others
* persistent, inconsolable grief

Creatively, people with excess Metal tend to be rigid and extremely neat, tending toward precise endeavors like architecture or medical illustration. They are perfectionists also, but of a more exacting type than those with Metal deficiency—Metal-excess folks require that everything look neat. Sometimes, their need for neatness prevents Metal-excess people from engaging in creative activity at all—they're afraid of the chaos, and unwilling to undertake something that may not come out perfect.

When Metal excess is the primary imbalance, the other elements may do the following:

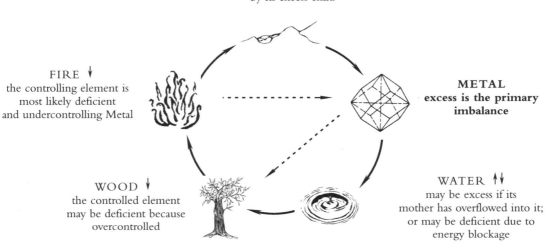

EARTH ↓
Metal's mother may be
deficient, because drained
by its excess child

FIRE ↓
the controlling element is
most likely deficient
and undercontrolling Metal

METAL
**excess is the primary
imbalance**

WOOD ↓
the controlled element
may be deficient because
overcontrolled

WATER ↑↓
may be excess if its
mother has overflowed into it;
or may be deficient due to
energy blockage

Luisa W. came to acupuncture for treatment of rheumatoid arthritis. She complained of pain and stiffness in many joints, but was particularly bothered by pain in the thumb and forefinger on both hands. Luisa also complained of a skin disorder that caused her to break out in patches of itchy, red, and dry skin. Luisa's face was pale, and her skin overall lacked luster.

Luisa's complaints correspond to a pattern of Metal excess, which overcontrols Wood and drains Earth. The Metal excess is discernible in the location of Luisa's most immediate pain: The thumb and forefinger are traversed by the Lung and Large Intestine meridians. The skin disorder indicates Metal involvement as

well. (When asked whether she had ever suffered from asthma or any kind of lung problems, Luisa reported that as a baby she had sometimes stopped breathing, and that her father was frequently required to give mouth-to-mouth resuscitation to revive her. Although such lung involvement is not necessary to diagnose a Metal imbalance, it is not surprising either.)

Arthritis is a disease with many contributing factors, but its stiffness and tendency to wander from joint to joint indicate Wood issues. In Luisa's case, swelling and some joint deformation also indicate phlegm—an Earth imbalance. Metal thus appears to be overcontrolling Wood and draining Earth, causing symptoms in both of those elements. Finally, the dry, itchy skin and pale, lusterless complexion indicate a blood deficiency. In Luisa's case, this would be the result of combined Earth and Wood deficiencies, which are responsible for building and nourishing Blood.

A special case of Metal excess occurs when we catch a cold or flu. In this instance, our own Metal defensive qi is weak and deficient, leaving room for a pathogenic wind from outside the body to invade. The invading pathogen creates signs of excess in the body, even though our own qi is actually deficient. Invasion by a pathogenic wind can result in

* runny nose

* achy muscles—particularly around the shoulders and back of the head

* a swollen or scratchy throat

* chills or an aversion to wind

* fever

Autumn swept the grasses and their color changed; she met the trees, and their boughs were stripped.

And because Autumn's being is compounded or sternness, therefore it was that they withered and perished, fell and decayed.

—Ou-yang Hsiu

METAL AND ACUPUNCTURE

When acupuncture uses metal needles or electrical current to stimulate the points and meridians, it calls upon Metal energies. In addition, practitioners use the Five Element points illustrated below to influence Metal's role in the Five Element cycle.

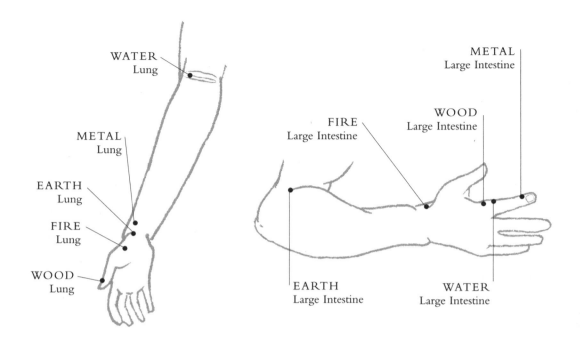

The Five Element Points on the
Lung Meridian

The Five Element Points on the
Large Intestine Meridian

The **Wood** points on the Metal meridians are used primarily to affect the relationship between Metal and Wood, the element it controls. Metal points would be tonified when the Wood element is excess and backing up into Metal, for instance, causing symptoms like a stuffy feeling in the chest and shortness of breath.

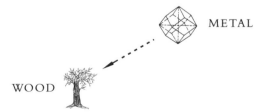

The **Fire** points on the Metal meridians are used to adjust Fire's level of control over the Metal element. When Metal is in excess, Fire points would be tonified to help it control Metal. These points would be dispersed, however, to relax Fire's control if Metal were deficient.

FIRE   METAL

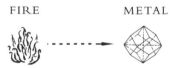

The **Earth** points on the Metal meridians are commonly tonified to strengthen Metal through its mother in the creation cycle.

EARTH

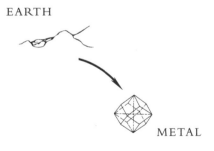

METAL

The **Metal** points on the Metal meridians have an extra ability to affect the Metal element—to strengthen it in deficiency and to disperse it when in excess. They are also commonly used whenever Metal's powers are needed—

to help tonify its child, Water, for instance, or to control an overactive Wood.

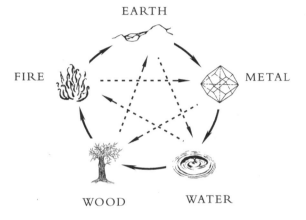

The **Water** points on Metal meridians affect Metal's relationship with Water, and can be dispersed to drain Metal excess through its child, or tonified to strengthen the child so it doesn't drain its deficient mother.

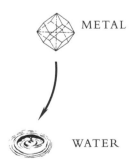

METAL

WATER

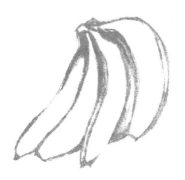

METAL AND FOOD

The Metal element manifests in food as the pungent flavor, root vegetables, fruits with thick peels, and the color white. In addition, the kinds of foods eaten during Metal's season—autumn—also affect its overall health. Metal's foods can be used in a variety of ways to help influence Metal's dynamic in the Five Element cycle.

Metal's flavor: pungence

Pungence is a Yang flavor that disperses energy and stimulates the body, moving energy upward and outward. These actions mimic Fire, the element that controls Metal, and can therefore control an overactive Metal element.

Because it is stimulating, pungence balances Metal's Yin propensity to stagnate. Pungent foods penetrate the Lung and Large Intestine, where they can be used in combination with other foods to affect various disorders in those organs. Pungent foods are generally divided into two categories—those that are warming and those that are cooling. Warming pungents include garlic and onions, chili peppers, horseradish, fennel, anise, dill, mustard greens, cinnamon, nutmeg, basil, rosemary, scallions, cloves, ginger, black pepper, and cayenne. Cooling pungents include radishes, cabbage, marjoram, white pepper, taro root, and turnip. Pungent herbs include citrus peel, ginger, and bupleurum.

Metal's vegetables: roots and tubers

Roots grow downward into the soil and thus embody Metal's internalizing and deepening properties. Some examples of root vegetables are potatoes, yams, turnips, carrots, radishes, ginger, garlic, and onion. Many of the root vegetables are also pungent, but their rootedness is another Metal quality. They are best eaten to strengthen Metal deficiencies, or to support Metal during the autumn.

Metal's fruits:
those that need to be peeled

Fruits with thick peels—like citrus fruits, bananas, and mangoes—are like the refined essences that Metal creates. The fruit is the pure essence that remains after the excess skin is discarded. Many of these fruits are also potent diuretics, which further illustrates their Metal and draining properties. Metal fruits are highly eliminative and best eaten to strengthen Metal deficiencies and to control excess Wood. They should not be eaten too freely in autumn, however, as they are raw and chilling at a time when foods should be warming.

Metal's color: white

Metal's white foods include onions, garlic, cauliflower, turnips, and parsnips. They are good for strengthening Metal deficiencies and for autumn diets.

Dispersing Metal Excess

Pungent foods are most often used to control Metal excess because they imitate Fire. If a Metal excess occurs with signs of Fire, however, like a fever, inflammation, or yellow or green phlegm, it is important to be careful with the pungent foods that are also warming (garlic, onions, chilis, ginger, and clove). In regulated amounts, these foods can push heat to the surface and clear it out through sweating, but in larger amounts they will exacerbate heat conditions.

Other foods to eat during times of Metal excess are Water foods, which help to drain their mother's excess. Dryness conditions can be helped by eating moistening foods like soybean products, spinach, barley, pears, apples, seaweeds, dairy products, shellfish, and honey.

Tonifying Metal Deficiency: Food and Autumn

A diet for autumn, or any other time when Metal needs to be supported, should be hearty and rich. Metal's root vegetables are perfect foods for cool autumn and winter months, helping

RECIPE FOR A WIND INVASION
A special case of Metal excess

Wind invasions are a special category of Metal excess discussed earlier, which can be easily dispersed with pungent foods if they are caught in the early stages. At the first sign of a cold or flu—sore or scratchy throat, or upper back, neck, or headache, take a hot bath or shower and enjoy the following soup.

Boil 2 cloves of garlic, fresh ginger, a radish, and scallions for 15 minutes in water or a light soup stock, then drink 3 to 4 times a day on an empty stomach. Often this soup will cause sweating, which is a sign that the pathogen is being pushed out of the body. Other ways to help get rid of a cold or flu in its earliest stages are hot baths and showers, head and neck massages, and peppermint or chamomile tea with a pinch of cayenne. Don't overeat, as a focus on digestion inhibits the body's ability to fight off pathogenic winds.

RECIPE FOR METAL DEFICIENCY
Onion and Cauliflower Curry

This flavorful dish encourages Metal's drying functions and adds a warm touch to autumn's chill. Its pungent spices, white vegetables, and dry texture all support Metal's functions.

1 head of cauliflower, cut into small florets

1 stalk of celery, cleaned and cut into $\frac{1}{4}$-inch pieces

6 tbsp. grapeseed or olive oil

2 medium onions, diced

5 cloves garlic, minced

2 tsp. pureed fresh ginger

$\frac{1}{2}$ small hot chili pepper, diced

Spice Mixture

2 tsp. ground cumin seeds

1 tsp. ground black mustard seeds

1 tsp. ground coriander seed

1 tsp. turmeric

$\frac{1}{2}$ tsp. ground fennel seeds

$\frac{1}{2}$ tsp. sea salt

4 fresh tomatoes, diced

$\frac{1}{4}$ cup water

1. Steam the cauliflower and celery for 8 to 1o minutes, or until soft.

2. While the vegetables are steaming, heat the oil in a large skillet and sauté the onion until it is clear.

3. Add the garlic, ginger, and chili pepper and cook for 1 minute.

4. Add the spices and stir-fry for an additional minute.

5. Add the tomatoes and the water, cooking for 1 to 2 minutes until the tomatoes are soft. Add the celery and cauliflower, stirring them thoroughly into the spiced mixture. If necessary, add more water to keep the dish from burning and cook for 2 minutes. Serve promptly.

to consolidate and lower body energy (like sap) so that it doesn't become too dispersed. Stronger-tasting and heartier foods, as well as longer cooking methods help to support this process. More meats, nuts, fish, and oils are appropriate, as are long cooking methods like baking and roasting, which draw abundant heat energy into foods to keep us warmer during colder months.

Bitter and salty foods, too, draw energy inward and downward, and should be used with increasing frequency as the weather gets cooler.

METAL AND QIGONG

The Metal element is an important part of QiGong practice, which uses many breathing exercises to affect the movement and overall quality of qi, as well as to reaffirm our connection with the Heavens.

Through the breath, Metal connects us to the qi of the universe and helps to produce qi in the body. Whereas the Earth element absorbs the qi of the universe through the ingestion of very solid Earthly substances, Metal brings in the more ethereal aspect of qi. Our

Lungs inhale Heaven's qi and transmute it, with the fires of our own essence, into a refined and nourishing body qi. This qi is pumped into every cell in our bodies, where it activates and vitalizes our basic life processes. With exhalation we eliminate byproducts and waste, which rejoin the celestial qi in the heavens and go on to nourish the vegetable kingdom. This simple exchange describes the very essence of the relationship; its profound poetry reminds us that we are intermingled with all of life.

In fact, the rhythm of our breath echoes the primal rhythm of the universe, demonstrating that we are but a microcosm of its grand design. Indeed, the rising and setting of the sun and moon, the ebb and flow of ocean tides, the contraction and expansion of a heartbeat, and the beckoning and thrust of sexual connection all tap out life's primal beat, amplifying a rhythm they contain but do not create. YinYang is one way of describing this fundamental rhythm; QiGong breathing practices are a way of bringing our minds and bodies into harmony with it.

There are many different kinds of breathing practiced in QiGong, and they have varying functions intended to regulate, promote, and direct the body's energy and essence in specific ways. A few of these practices are discussed below, but the reader is encouraged to consult sourcebooks listed in the References section for more information, and to try some QiGong or Yoga classes.

Normal breathing

The most basic QiGong breathing practice is called "normal breathing." It challenges us to become aware of our fundamental breathing patterns. In normal breathing one simply pays attention to the process of breathing without striving to control it or change it in any way. What we become aware of when we become aware of breathing is the action of our lungs, diaphragm, and stomach muscles, our noses and mouths, lips and teeth. The lungs themselves can neither expand nor contract; it's the action of the diaphragm sinking and the stomach muscles expanding that draw breath into the lungs, and their subsequent rise and contraction that forces air back out again. In becoming aware of this process, we are reminded of the very physical nature of being.

In addition, we become aware of the quality of our breath. Whether it flows in and out smoothly or roughly, evenly or in fits and starts, loudly or quietly, fully or partially, deeply or

EXERCISE: NORMAL BREATHING

To do normal breathing, sit quietly and calmly with a straight back, on a chair or a firm cushion on the floor. Close your eyes and just pay attention. It is often difficult for beginners to focus their minds on breath, and many find that they have to keep reining their thoughts in. It may be helpful to count during breathing—from one to ten and then backward from ten to one, repeating the cycle for five or ten minutes or as long as the breathing exercise lasts. Don't count the breaths themselves, just count—as slowly or as quickly as seems comfortable and enough to keep your thoughts from wandering.

shallowly, etc. This clues us in to the state of our emotions and well-being; whether we're calm or agitated, distracted or focused, sleepy or aware, and so on.

The purpose of normal breathing is to focus awareness on the breath in order to tune in to the current state of the body and the primal hum of the universe.

Abdominal breathing

Abdominal breathing is the next step in the breathing practice; it teaches us to expand our lungs more fully in order to draw in more fresh energy from

EXERCISE: ABDOMINAL BREATHING

When doing abdominal breathing, one should sit quietly and comfortably, with a straight back. First do normal breathing to center and focus the mind, and to tune in to the various organs involved in breathing. Slowly move the focus of your breath downward from the chest into the abdomen. You may want to put one hand on your belly so you can feel it expand and contract. The belly should expand as you inhale; this draws air into the lungs via suction. At the same time, the diaphragm sinks downward, allowing the lungs to expand more fully. With exhalation, the shoulders drop, the chest sinks inward, the diaphragm rises, and the belly should contract gently and easily. This pushes the stale air out through the lungs. Do this breath for two or three minutes, keeping focus on the abdomen and diaphragm, trying to relax and expand them more and more.

At the same time, try to notice the quality of the breath. It should be silent and smooth, without ratchety stops and starts. Inhalation and exhalation should flow continuously into each other without pauses, and they should be equal in length or longer on exhalation. When you notice unevenness in your quality of breath, just try to keep relaxing. Don't force smoothness, but let it come naturally as your breaths get deeper and deeper.

the cosmos, and to exhale more completely in order to clear stale energy out. Abdominal breathing uses the muscles of the abdomen to pull down the diaphragm, which then draws air into the lungs. Most adults tend to breathe exclusively from their chests, which does not render a full breath.

In practicing abdominal breathing, one achieves many effects. More oxygen comes into the body, which nourishes tissues and organs. The heart slows and steadies, which calms the mind and the spirit. More clear qi is refined and distributed, meaning more is available to the body, and more is able to be stored as essence.

Yin Yang breathing

YinYang breathing is a breath that balances the right and left sides of the body, the Yin and Yang functions, and the nervous system. In Yoga it is known as alternate-nostril breathing. As with other breathing exercises, this one begins with a comfortable seated position, a straight back, and a few minutes of normal breathing to calm and focus the mind.

Ideally, this breath can be combined with abdominal breathing to ensure maximum expansion of the Lungs. It should be smooth, quiet, and regular, with exhalations lasting up to twice as long as inhalations. This is a good

EXERCISE: YINYANG BREATHING

Make a loose fist with the index and middle fingers of the right hand, leaving the thumb and the last two fingers extended. Using the ring and pinky fingers, gently close off the left nostril and breathe deeply in through the right. As you reach the top of your inhalation, release the left nostril and close off the right one with your thumb. Exhale slowly and smoothly. At the end of exhalation, breathe in deeply through the uncovered left nostril. When this inhalation is complete, open the right nostril and close the left one again with the last two fingers, exhaling deeply and slowly through the right nostril before beginning the cycle all over again. Continue this exercise for two to four minutes.

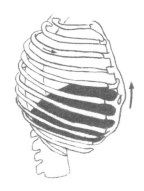

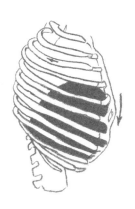

During inhalation, the diaphragm contracts and creates suction, which draws in air through the lungs (above top). During exhalation, the diaphragm expands to push air back out (above bottom).

breath to practice first thing in the morning, to balance the body and mind in preparation for the day ahead. If your left nostril remains congested or clogged throughout the exercise, it may be an early sign of a wind invasion: It would be a good idea to drink the Metal-excess soup described on page 154.

Many other breathing exercises help to direct qi to specific organs, to heighten mental awareness, and to activate or sedate qi energy. Over time, these breathing practices calm the mind and heal the body by renewing our relationship with the rhythms of the universe.

METAL AND FENG SHUI

Metal's qualities of separation and refinement manifest in the environment as metal objects, machinery, electronics, and rounded surfaces. Metal also governs the vast network of calculations that measure and define our natural world—the math that informs physics, geometry, astrology, astronomy, and other sciences. These calculations quantify the interactions of Heaven and Earth using Metal's faculties of discerning and separating.

In China, such calculations have classically been performed with the Feng Shui compass, which provides information about cosmological and terralogical forces pertaining to a particular site. A complicated assembly of up to thirty-eight rings or tiers, the compass has long been a tool for the most skilled and educated practitioners. It can be categorized as belonging to the Metal element for two reasons: because it is magnetic and therefore relies on Metal energies to function, and because the complex sorting and dividing that the various tiers employ is an aspect of Metal's function of separation.

The innermost rings usually describe the eight trigrams of the Ba–Gua, and thereby the cardinal and intracardinal points. Other tiers help to pinpoint the most powerful spots at a particular site, to determine the optimal site for a burial, the optimal time to begin building, or the quality of the watercourses. Some tiers are connected to the angles of the sun in the sky, others to the positions of the stars, others to magnetic currents in the ground or to various divinatory systems. Some tiers are directly connected to the Five Element cycle, while others correspond to the complex Chinese calendar.

Outdoors, the Metal element corresponds to mountains that are rounded and oblong, and to buildings that have rounded or domed roofs. Arches with their rounded tops also invoke Metal.

Indoors, Metal shapes are rounded and sinking like pillows and hassocks, globes and knobs. They can also look like truncated Fire shapes as in cone-shaped lampshades.

Metal colors are white and metallic. The best color for a kitchen, white is compatible with the Fire that rules there. Metal and white in a kitchen encourage Fire to increase and control them, although red

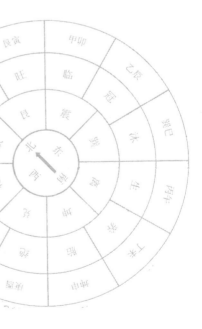

Feng Shui Compass

kitchens create too much Fire. Metal materials are metals like silver, brass, copper, and gold as well as mirrored surfaces. Jewelry, watches, and crystals are also aligned with the Metal element.

Mirrors are a popular Feng Shui tool and can be used to balance energy anywhere it has gone awry. Mirrors can be hung facing outdoors to deflect the overbearing energy of nearby neighbors, mountains, or buildings. (Convex mirrors are especially fun for this purpose, as they will reflect the mountain or building back to itself upside down!) They can also be hung so as to bring the image of nearby water (pond or river) into the house to encourage prosperity.

Mirrors are useful hung on walls or in corners that trap or stop qi flow—like a wall that interrupts your sight line when you enter a room, or a recessed corner. They can help to rectify an oddly shaped room or cure a badly placed stove or bed. Mirrors are one of the basic cures used by Feng Shui practitioners, and can adjust a wide variety of Feng Shui maladies.

Electric and particularly electronic devices also manifest Metal energies, as they are produced from metal parts—wires, connectors, and silicon chips. Like mirrors, they can be used to bring energy and movement to any stagnating area.

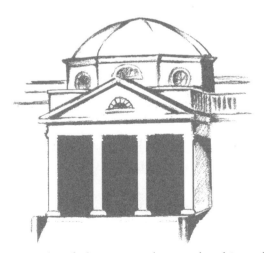

Domed roofs draw energy downward and inward, invoking Metal's consolidating functions.

Tonifying Metal Deficiency

Adding Metal to tonify a deficiency can be best accomplished by cleaning. Sweeping, vacuuming, washing, and scrubbing are guaranteed ways to eliminate unnecessary dirt and bring out some refined essence. People who clean compulsively overuse this mechanism in an effort to get "pure" of some imagined or imposed taint, but when it's undertaken appropriately, cleaning can help Metal regain its purification and separation functions.

In addition, one can add new decorative pillows to a couch or chair (preferably white), hang a new mirror in a prominent place, or repaint the walls with a fresh, clean white. Wear white, metal, or crystals to deflect and squeeze out unwanted thoughts, worries, or obsessions. As white is the color of cleansing and purification, wear it to let go of unwanted ideas or oppressive griefs.

Other ways to strengthen deficient Metal involve adding Earth elements as described in the Earth chapter, and reducing Fire.

Dispersing Metal Excess

To control a Metal excess, it's important to enrich your surroundings. If Metal has overpurified, the first rule of thumb is to add—add color, shape, sound, texture, and especially smell. Since Metal rules the sense of smell, fragrances are a joyful way to stimulate it, via incense, perfumes, flowers, and home cooking.

All the senses will benefit from enrichment, however, so take a luxurious bath with fragrant oils, hang up some new, colorful artwork, play music, watch movies, wear your softest silk or cotton pajamas.

In addition, add Fire to control excess Metal, and Water to drain it.

Note, however, that the special case of Metal excess marked by a cold or flu ought not to be treated with these Metal-excess strategies in Feng Shui. They should be treated, instead, by the Metal deficiency Feng Shui suggestions, which will help to eliminate the pathogen.

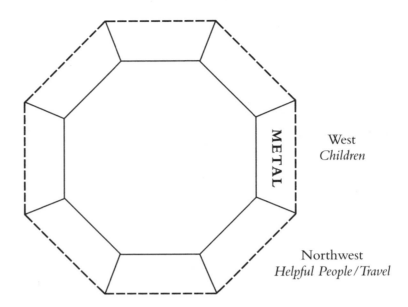

METAL

West
Children

Northwest
Helpful People/Travel

The Metal area of the Ba-Gua is the west, which also corresponds to children. To rectify a Metal element imbalance, place a mirror on a western wall, hang a prism or crystal, or place a metal candle holder or wall sconce. Alternatively, a computer, stereo, or other electronic device is well placed on a western wall.

The northwest corresponds to helpful people and travel: northwest walls and corners are therefore good places to store globes, maps, and telephone books. Hang mirrors or crystals in this area of the living room or study to promote interaction with helpful people and new places.

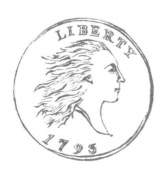

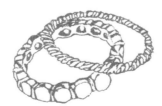

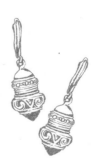

22

*It's possible I am pushing through solid rock
in flintlike layers, as the ore lies, alone;
I am such a long way in I see no way through,
and no space: everything is close to my face,
and everything close to my face is stone.*

*I don't have much knowledge yet in grief—
so this massive darkness makes me small.
You be the master: make yourself fierce, break in:
then your transforming will happen to me,
and my great grief cry will happen to you.*

—Rainer Maria Rilke

A balanced Metal element allows us to move beyond the situations that disappoint us, cutting through pain and grief to isolate the wisdom each experience holds. We recognize that loss is a part of life and do not cling to what is no longer within our grasp. Healthy Metal keeps us present in the moment, focusing our accumulated wisdom to help us make the judgments that will determine our life's trajectory.

As Metal's process of separation approaches completion, the pure becomes recognizably distinct from the impure, and our newly acquired wisdom becomes distinct from the circumstances that catalyzed it. Once such separation is complete, it's time to take a step back and integrate our new wisdom into the larger context of our being. This greater context is the Water element, which subsumes distilled essence as well as that which was discarded from it, maintaining a setting in which both belong. Water remains whole regardless of what is purified or separated within its infinite boundary. It is where we reconnect with our innermost selves and allow new experiences to move us one step further along our destined paths.

WATER

CHAPTER 6

WATER SYMBOLIZES BOTH LIFE AND DEATH: IT IS the womb from which all life emerges and the abyss to which it returns. As the universal oneness that exists beyond and within all individuals, water is similar to the Tao itself. Though separate lives coalesce out of its unity, they are like drops of water temporarily distinct from the sea; it is only a matter of time before they rejoin their eternal whole.

Many mythologies (Greek, Chinese, Mesopotamian) describe the birth of humankind as a watery event, initiated by the semen of a god that fell into the oceans, by the mating of the sun and moon, whose raindrops fell into the oceans, or by the product of two islands in the ocean, among other tales. In these stories water is the womb that gives birth to us all.

Like the womb, water engenders birth, and is used as an agent of renewal in ritual baths, baptisms, and libations. The womb's watery suspension also represents a kind of nonexistence, however, as a timeless, spaceless interlude in which we hold no awareness of self or world. This ocean of peace is the same void we return to when we die, and it is thus that water comes to represent death as well as birth.

In death, water marks the ceasing of individual form and consciousness. While the waters of Lethe cause us to forget, rivers often form a border between life and death. Those who "cross over" the river Styx, for instance, are on their way to the land of the dead—often in the care of a boatman who is a messenger between the worlds. Bodies of water often serve as such portals between the ordinary world of human beings and the Otherworlds of death or faerie. Water's magical creatures—ladies of the lake, nymphs, mermaids, selkies, etc.—all have the potential for tremendous magic, which can give or take life.

Water itself acts as an agent of death, whose torrents, floods, and tempests have destroyed many a civilization from Atlantis to Noah's biblical home. Whereas Fire destroys by dispersion, Water completely subsumes, annihilating all form in its deep belly. In this vengeful aspect Water wreaks a destruction more total than that of any other force, reminding us that the void is the most terrible power of all.

Even our most mundane encounters with water remind us of other states of being. When calm like a still pool, water stands for absolute tranquillity— a state as boundless as the void whose image it evokes. When channeled in steady motion, water symbolizes the patience of eternity—as when a single drop carves canyons out of stone, or the ocean rolls by in perpetual tides. Water's quiet endurance knows no temporal limit.

Water in the Five Element cycle includes these

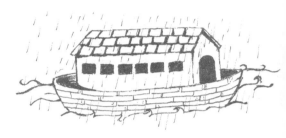

Water's powers of total annihilation are evident in the world's many tales of cataclysmic flooding.

aspects of life, death, and eternity. It signifies the culmination of process—completion and death—and it portends renewal. Both destructive and creative, the Water element serves as a bridge between life and death, and between death and rebirth. It governs a state of limbo between worlds, and as such signifies a pause, a gulf, or a void. Water's action is nonaction and its form is no-form, like the great Tao whose essence it echoes. In physics, Water corresponds to an object at rest, containing all potential and no kinetic energy.

Water is the child of Metal in the Creation cycle. As the runoff created by Metal's distillation, Water signifies wholeness, for it is a medium that integrates even the waste discarded by others. It remains as whole when something has been added to it as when something has been completely removed from it. As explained by one of Zen Buddhism's ancient masters, Eihei Dogen, "Water is the only truth of water. Water is water's complete virtue."

Water is controlled by Earth, which dams it, pools it, and thereby contains its formlessness. In the YinYang cycle, Water represents absolute Yin—absolute rest, passivity, and receptivity.

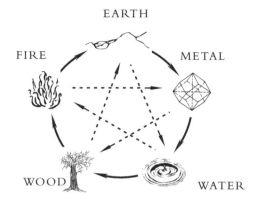

Without a shape of its own, water pools in whatever indentations it falls into, joining itself instantly like a drop in a puddle or merging completely into the ground. In the Water phase, individual objects and processes similarly forgo their unique identities to merge with the great pool of the Tao, returning to the universal soup from which they sprang. Whether this return is achieved through quiet release or chaotic destruction makes no difference; Water takes by any means necessary.

Water as a season corresponds with winter, a period of rest and restoration. Winter's dark hours and cold temperatures manifest this season's absolute Yin, as does the sharp quiet peculiar to winter nights. The hush of a silent snowfall makes Water's tranquillity almost palpable, as voices sink into whispers and footsteps fall into muted silence.

Trees stand dormant in winter, their roots and branches sleeping until the spring's sun brings them to life again, while hibernating animals also enter long, deep sleeps that are scarcely broken by their infrequent breaths. Winter's cold minimizes activity and stalls growth, as plants and animals conserve their resources in preparation for the season's harsher times. Evidence of life is not completely lacking, just in hiding as living things conserve their potential in storage rather than in open manifestation.

This period of storage is vital, as it allows the organism to rest and repair from its long seasons of activity. Just as humans consult their dreams during sleep for visions of their source and potential, so do plants and animals commune with their deepest potential during winter's dormancy. Without this "dead of winter" there would be no life to spring.

In the cycle of a day, Water governs night and sleep. At night, most people and businesses lie dormant, restoring their energies for the new day. At this time our tissues, cells, and organs rest in a state of reduced activity that engenders repair. Although modern sleep scientists don't understand why we sleep, it's an inevitable occurrence from the point of view of the Five Element system: The dormancy of sleep epitomizes the Water phase, and so is crucial to the continuation of days. We fall into sleep as surely as Metal generates Water—habitually, regularly, and needfully—and we emerge from it just as regularly, into the periods of activity that manifest the Wood phase. We sleep, therefore, for the same reason that

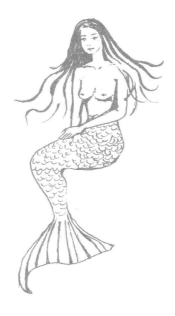

Mermaids and other mythical Water beings are symbols of freedom and imagination; many of their stories describe how they become trapped in earth's mundane reality and lose their creative powers.

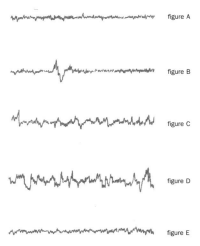

figure A

figure B

figure C

figure D

figure E

During Water's sleeping and dreaming states, brainwaves show varying patterns. The dream state (REM sleep) in figure E shows calm brainwaves that are characteristic of dreaming's active imagination.

there's darkness between sunset and sunrise: because Water's abyss claims everything between completion and new beginning.

Dreaming is a Watery phenomenon, linked with sleep, that invokes Water's merging of all boundaries as well as its infinite imagination. Dreams take us out of the world as we know it and locate us in a strange and formless universe, where time and space have no hold, and where knowledge is instantaneous and omnipotent. In dreams we connect to the universal mind, the great Tao, whose wisdom and prophesy often comes to us in sleep. Our dreams give us glimpses of the universal whole, and serve as powerful guides and teachers throughout our lives.

Like dreaming, reverie is a Water activity that takes us out of the regular world and into a deeper realm. Less concrete than memory, reverie is a waking dream, an inward sea without time or space boundaries, where we float, connecting to the experiences that give us meaning. Such daydreaming reminds us that we are larger than the reality to which we are bound, and thus evokes the world-beyond-the-edges where Water resides.

In the construction of a building, Water time begins when the building is completed. The workers have gone home, and the building lies silent and empty—perhaps humming with electricity and heat, getting ready for its inhabitants, but not yet inhabited. Lying dormant, the building stands in preparation for beginning the cycle again. Although the construction project is dead, the building is just coming to life, where it will begin a whole new existence.

Water is the source of creativity governing the formlessness out of which new ideas cohere. It is a space without boundaries, and thus the haven where imagination thrives. Artists of all kinds draw their sustenance from Water's freedom and may feel more at home there than in ordinary reality. Such people are often called eccentric because they spend so much time in worlds of their own—and Water's—making. Creativity dwells in Watery realms because that's where anything can happen—the only limits are those imposed by our own shortsightedness.

During the course of any specific project, Water is the tap from which ideas spring; it is the source of creative possibilities, surrounding individual projects and serving as the context in which they are created. It also marks the end of every project, however, that moment of separation when the activity is done and there is no more "project" to speak of. In the abyss of completion one may step back and admire the work that was done, envision its use and display, or walk away and take a nap. Any and all of

these are appropriate activities in the Water phase; the only thing that can't be done is more work.

Marcia O., a screenwriter and director, was listless for months after finishing her first film, sleeping long hours, window shopping, and reading novels, but growing increasingly angry at herself for not beginning her next project. Marcia felt that she was being lazy, and she wondered what was causing this downtime that she perceived as a creative block. She didn't understand that downtime was necessary, however, and that Water was demanding rest in exact proportion to the amount of effort she had expended in her work. This is always the case with Water, and no amount of wishing or trying can rush its restorative process.

What Marcia didn't realize at the time was that while all this "nothing" was going on, she was deeply engaged on her innermost levels with Water's creative energies. When she did finally come up with an idea for a new project, it was one that excited her tremendously. In her new Wood phase, hard at work on her new script, Marcia better understood the nature of the quietude she had just experienced.

In the natural world, Water's ultimate creativity is vital to the survival of every living thing. It forms the oceans from which all life emerged and fills the wombs that nurture us into life. Ninety-eight percent of our bodily substance is composed of water, which also hangs in the air we breathe and vitalizes the foods we eat. Water is so much a part of life that life cannot long exist without it; it inheres in the animal, vegetable, and mineral kingdoms, echoing the enormous presence of the Tao as the source of all.

In cosmology, Water corresponds to the condition of unity that existed before the Big Bang, as well as a hypothetical return to that oneness when the universe dies. Whether physicists describe this condition as a "singularity" or a point of "infinite density,"* it is scarcely different from the cosmic whole that has inspired mystics through the ages. As the Great Mystery, the Dreamtime, the formless void, primordial chaos, or the Tao, oneness is the state of the primordial universe, and a profound image of the Water element.

In the menstrual cycle, Water time is menstruation—the bleeding of "heavenly water" that cleanses the womb of dead cells and leaves it ready to begin the fertility cycle again. All cultures associate menstruation with the moon, whose twenty-eight day revolution around the earth coincides with the length of the average menstrual cycle. The moon thus controls the tides of menstruation as it does ocean tides, inciting peaks and hollows (ovulation and menstruation) with its own waxing and waning. In fact, the words "month," "moon," and "menses" all derive from the same ancient root, and many traditions describe the fertility cycle as a "moon cycle."

Some Chinese traditions call menstrual blood the "red snow," an appellation which plainly connects it to the Water element and its season. In many cultures, menstruating women accommodate the Water phase of their cycles by removing themselves from everyday activity to spend time with other women in meditation, artwork, and storytelling. They celebrate the altered consciousness of the Water state by communing with the Great Mystery

* Stephen Hawking, "The Edge of Spacetime."

of their inner selves, their creativity, and their gods.

In modern Western culture, few lives will allow for such complete withdrawal on a regular basis. However, most women recognize the need for it, craving rest, warm foods, and soothing experiences without fully understanding that these are the very things required by the body and the soul. Water time calls for rest, introversion, and a recognition of the sacredness of existence—when we meet it with the same old daily grind we may find ourselves weepy, irritable, and frustrated by menstrual tension of all kinds. Many women find they have fewer difficulties with their periods when they learn to "go with the flow" of their moon cycles, abandoning their daily routine to allow their bodies and minds a glimpse of a more universal existence.

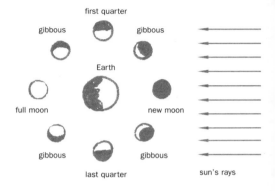

Phases of the moon

*The forces of winter create
cold in Heaven and water on Earth.
They create the kidney organ
and the bones within the body . . .
the emotion fear, and the ability to
make a groaning sound.*

—The Yellow Emperor's Classic of Internal Medicine

The climate that corresponds to Water is cold. Cold is a Yin force that contracts, slows, and reduces both mass and movement. Cold water, winter air, ice cream, air conditioners, ocean currents, and dark forests are some of the places we encounter cold in our daily lives.

Cold brings stillness, silence, and rest to organisms that would otherwise burn themselves out. It tempers heat by calming its restless activity. In summer, the cool earth and cold waters protect plants and animals from the sun's parching and burning. Cool nights bring respite from scorching days, as cool breezes do likewise in suffocating heat.

Too much cold, however, extinguishes vitality altogether. It causes damage by inhibiting movement so that growth is stunted and extremities die from lack of nourishment. When the water of life is frozen solid, life itself ceases.

In the body as in nature, cold allows for repair: It slows movement, giving cells an opportunity to restore what they've lost so that they can continue their normal processes. Without cold's tempering influence, we would all die much sooner, burning out our organs from overactivity. Too much cold, though, causes its own problems in the body—it inhibits digestion and can give rise to loose stool, belching, and abdominal pain, while in the joints it inhibits

movement, causing pain and stiffness.

Environmentally, cold describes influences that are lacking or deficient in some way, as opposed to the "too much of" condition that is heat. Indoor lighting is deficient because it lacks full-spectrum energies, while processed food is deficient because it lacks the vital qi and vitamins we need.

Water on an emotional level governs inner strength. It is the source of such strength as it is the source of creativity—existing beneath our conscious awareness as a wellspring from which we draw. Water's power is not about action, or even preparation for action, but the power of potential action that we hold within. On a daily level, Water energy governs our awareness of our internal resources. It gives us the knowledge that we will be able to handle whatever life brings. Water grants us equanimity, and the confidence that comes with knowing we have what we need.

Many people do not know the full measure of their strength until they have been tested in some way—until some crisis taps the courage they didn't know they had. It is the Water element that stores these hidden strengths, and brings them into play when they are most needed.

Implicit in the Chinese understanding of internal resources is the idea of a spiritual or ancestral strength: We all contain the strengths of our ancestors in addition to our individual powers. What's more, we can draw upon their strength when our own fails us. Many cultures around the world raise their children to understand that they are parts of a continuous whole, which stretches through them from the beginning of time to their children's children and beyond. This notion of unity beyond the borders of the individual is Water energy in its grandest sense. It describes strength through knowledge of the profound continuity of life in the universe.

But while knowing one's strengths is the positive manifestation of internal Water energy, its negative side is fear— the emotion associated with Water in classical Chinese medicine. Fear happens when we doubt our strengths, when we feel alone and unconnected to the forces that support us, and therefore vulnerable to chaos or malevolence. Whether we're afraid of injury, of being judged, of death, or of confusion,

fear paralyzes us as completely as cold freezes. It stops us dead in our tracks, rendering us unable to pursue whatever audition, proposal, journey, or relationship was calling us forward into life and growth.

Most of us grow afraid when we feel ourselves extending beyond ordinary boundaries—in other words, when we enter Water's limitless territory. This commonly occurs when we're about to do something we have never done before—go skiing, perform in public, explore an unfamiliar place, etc. We may feel this fear contemplating actions as small as trying new food, or as big as fulfilling a portion of our destiny—whether the activity is likely to cause us actual harm or to bring us pleasure and enlightenment. Fear simply accompanies Water's unknown.

Some people feel fear in any situation they can't control—airplane rides, large groups of people, messy houses, visits to the doctor, etc. Such anxiety signals difficulty in surrendering to Water's uncontrollable void; those who suffer from it often cling to Metal's sharpened neuroses instead.

Chinese medicine sometimes distinguishes between fear and fright,

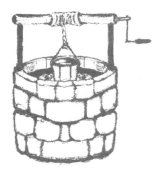

*Sources of fresh water,
like wells and streams,
often mark holy or
mystical sites. Such wells
act as portals to alternate
worlds and beings.*

describing fear as an internal fear of something, and fright as a sudden scare—a traumatic event like a car accident or a sinister shape leaping out of a dark corner. Both are governed by Water energy, and both affect one's ability to step forward into new situations in life; fright is simply considered a more acute condition than fear's long-standing habit.

We can learn to modulate Water's fear by developing inner resources we can trust. Reckoning honestly with our own strengths and weaknesses teaches us which aspects of our personality are dependable: These can be relied on in times of fear. For attributes we don't have, we learn that it's appropriate to apply to others for help. Although many people avoid asking for help out of embarrassment, it brings no shame if we have an accurate sense of our own strength. Instead, it teaches us to appreciate the gifts that other people have to give.

WATER IN THE
HUMAN LIFE CYCLE

In the human life cycle, Water rules death and dying, the period when we release our bodies to return to the oneness from which we came. Here we lose our individuated selves and, like a drop in the ocean, become one again with our great source.

In modern cultures, death is generally perceived with terror—Water's fear of its own unknown haunts us continually, crippling many lives. This fear has spawned the youth-obsessed culture that surrounds us, which denies age, wisdom, and death while fetishizing youth and inexperience. Fear of death also lies behind our most controversial legal issues—abortion rights, the death penalty, assisted suicide, and the right to die—as people and the courts struggle to define who should wield the power of life and death over someone else's body.

However, such consuming terror is not universal. Among people and in cultures where reincarnation or some sort of afterlife is assumed, death is quite clearly a stage in a cycle that renews itself continuously: Those who are reincarnated go around the wheel of life again and again. Under these conditions, death evokes less fear because it is less of an unknown quantity; people essentially know where they're going and what will be required of them when they get there.

Belief systems that disallow the renewal of the cycle, however, create an abyss at the end of life. It is terrifying because it is unknown, and people thus spend their entire lives fearing it. In terms of Five Element theory, such a permanent end does not make sense; Water by its very nature generates Wood, and death in this context leads inevitably to new life.

Stories abound of people all over the world who foresee their deaths long in advance and prepare themselves quietly and peacefully for that transitional event. Religious people and mystics of all kinds are known for such behavior. Indeed, *The Tibetan Book of Living and Dying* is a whole manual devoted to the mechanics of appropriate dying; it teaches us how to live and to die in the presence of our fears.

The spiritual aspect of Water is collectivity—our sense of being part of a whole. Collectivity invites us to feel connected not only to each other or to God, but to country, community, and the whole of creation—stars, sun, dust specks, insects, and the entire undulating universe. It gives us a larger sense of self, as it reminds us of the time before creation when we were all one.

Those who act with a consciousness of the greater good draw upon Water's collective spirit, understanding that the actions of one will affect all. Martyrs epitomize this collectivity: They sacrifice their own lives in an effort to improve the lives of others. This function of spirit is often abused by those in leadership positions, who convince their followers that sacrifice must be accomplished in order to benefit the greater whole. Suicide cults, kamikaze pilots, and the imperative to sacrifice luxuries during a "war effort" all tap Water's collective spirit in this way.

On a soul level, Water evokes destiny. Although we tend to think of destiny as our future, it has as much to do with our past; it is the thread that connects who we have been with who we will become. Just as the Tao is the whole from which individual beings separate, so destiny is the whole of one soul's journey, from which each moment and every lifetime temporarily individuates. It is the context in which we live our individual lives.

Destiny governs those attributes that we come into the world with: our original endowment of genes, family, and karma. These characteristics define who we are when we first begin life in the Wood phase: The choices we make every day determine what we will become as that original endowment is transformed by the events of our lives. The destiny that we approach during each lifetime creates for us the lessons, the experiences, the wisdom, and the power that will one day render us whole. The goal of life in the first place, wholeness is the reason we individuate: that we might learn to mirror the Tao that mirrors us all.

The Water element exists primarily outside of human relationships, more clearly invoking the relationship each individual has with his or her inner self. In the Water phase we examine our own inner knowledge, our dreams, our emotions, and all those aspects of our experience that can never be truly felt by another. It is less the imprint of experience on the self than it is the self that has the experience, remaining a constant entity throughout childhood, adulthood, friendships, romances, and working relationships.

Water governs who you are when your boss, lover, child, etc. leaves the room—what you reflect upon, agonize over, and dream about. While not itself about relationship, the Water phase is crucial to every connection. Without it, there is nobody there to relate to. In fact, our Watery selves are what we're in a relationship for: They prompt us to communicate who we are to the others in our lives.

Conversely, Water also gives us perspective on our relationships and our personal concerns. Because it bears a sense of the whole, Water allows us to step outside ourselves to visit our plans and circumstances from a different point of view. Water sees the context of things—the history, the dynamics, and the party politics of any given situation—thus affording us a more holistic understanding.

Water's vast perspective gives rise to compassion—the love and respect for others that arises from a sense of shared experience. Compassion is not the personal love associated with the Fire and Earth elements; it is more general, extending honor to all of creation simply because it exists. Compassion gives value to everything that lives. It does not pass judgment or collapse into pity, but loves deeply from a position of absolute respect. The more we cultivate compassion, the more conscious we become of our role in the greater whole.

WATER IN THE BODY

The Water element manifests in the body as the organs and meridians of the Kidneys (Yin) and the Bladder (Yang). Together, the Kidneys and Bladder govern the Water element's long perspective, internal sequestering, and peace. In addition, the organs of the Kidneys and Bladder have the following physiological functions.

The Kidneys are the source of all Yin and Yang in the body. The Kidneys are considered the "pilot light" that ignites the body's primary drives—Yin and Yang—and all the energy that is derived from their interaction. In this capacity, the Kidneys embody the Water element's function as the source of all. All the body's organs derive their stores of Yin and Yang— thus Water and Fire—from the Yin and Yang of the Kidneys.

Dysfunctions in this aspect of Kidney energy will result in deficiencies of Yin, Yang, or both.

The Kidneys store Essence. Essence, or jing, is a dense form of energy that gives substance and spark to an organism. It is produced in the Kidneys from a combination of inherited material (like DNA) and the refined essences of food and air. One of QiGong's Three Treasures, Essence can be understood as the physical form of the will to live. Seeking always to create (and procreate), Essence is the source of Water's infinite creativity.

Essence rules overall vitality and its strength determines the lifespan of every individual. It carries the body's inherited characteristics, including genes and karma, and also governs physical and sexual development, creating sexual secretions, sexual drive, and sexual function. When the Kidneys are unable to store Essence properly, a child may experience birth defects, mental retardation, or delayed development. If a Kidney imbalance occurs later in life, it can impair sexual drive and sexual function as well as a wide variety of other body functions. (See QiGong section on page 194 for more about Essence.)

The Kidneys rule the bones and teeth. Bones and teeth are the densest forms of matter in the body, and require large amounts of Kidney Essence for their development. The strength, integrity, and growth of the bones and teeth thus reflect the quality of Kidney energy available to the body. Malformed, weak, or decaying bones and teeth point to an imbalance in the Kidneys.

The Kidneys manifest in the head hair and open into the ears. The vitality of the Kidneys can be gauged from the quality of the head hair. Whether thick or thin, shiny or dull, oily or dry, richly colored or graying, hair's radiance reflects the radiance of the Kidneys and their Essence.

The ears and the sense of hearing also reflect the Kidneys. Problems like deafness, dizziness, and ringing in the ears can indicate a dysfunction of the Kidneys.

The Kidneys are also called the Kidney-Adrenal glands. Kidneys encompass the modern Western notion of adrenal glands as well as the whole endocrine system. Endocrine glands produce hormones, whose sexual and growth-catalysing properties are included in the descriptions of Kidney function.

The Kidneys grasp the qi from the Lungs. The Kidneys receive the air that the Lungs inhale and refine. This refined air is then used in the production of Kidney Yin, Kidney Yang, and Kidney Essence.

The Kidneys rule water. As the organs of the Water element, the Kidneys control the quality and quantity of urine. They also supply qi to the Bladder, which stores and eliminates urine. In addition, the Yang energy of the Kidneys helps the Small and Large Intestines to separate clean and dirty fluids, and provides the Spleen with the energy it needs to transform and transport fluids.

Imbalances in Kidney function can therefore be reflected in urinary tract diseases, incontinence, scanty or over-abundant urine, constipation, diarrhea, and phlegm diseases.

The Bladder stores and eliminates fluid waste. The Bladder receives Kidney qi and uses it to transform and eliminate fluids.

The Kidney and Bladder meridians manifest the Water element along the surface of the body. The Kidney meridian begins on the sole of the foot and travels up the inner aspect of the leg and groin, running up the trunk on either side of the midline to end just under the collarbone.

The Bladder meridian begins in the inner corner of the eye, goes around the head and down the back on either side

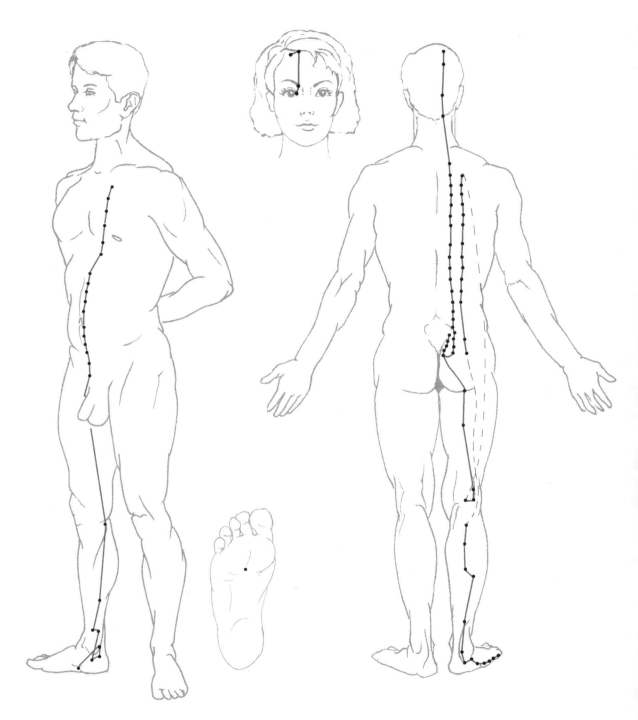

The Kidney Meridian   The Bladder Meridian

of the midline, to the back of the knee. It runs another line down the back alongside its previous line, which continues down the buttocks. Picking up again below the knee, the meridian travels along the back of the leg and the outer edge of the foot to end on the small toe.

WATER OUT OF BALANCE

Because the Kidneys are the source of the body's Essence and Yin and Yang energies, excesses rarely build up in them—one is never considered to have "too much" Essence. Most styles of acupuncture therefore hardly recognize Kidney or Water excesses—only various kinds of deficiency, which sometimes create an *appearance* of excess.

Water in Deficiency

Since the Water element is the source of Yin and Yang in the body, when it becomes deficient it can manifest as a deficiency of Yin or a deficiency of Yang. Each of these imbalances creates distinctive symptoms as follows.

Deficient Kidney Yin can be distinguished by:

* pain in the lower back and knees

* scanty, dark urine

* red tongue

* afternoon fevers

* malar flush (flushing of the cheeks but not the whole face)

* insomnia

* night sweats

* feelings of heat in the palms and soles

Other signs may include infertility, premature ejaculation, anxiety, hysteria, palpitations, prematurely gray hair, and feeling "tired and wired." On a creative level, deficient Kidney Yin usually manifests as an inability to attain the quietude required for entrance into Water's creative realm. People with deficient Kidney Yin are always wired—nervous and restless—and cannot relax fully enough to come up with creative ideas.

Deficient Kidney Yin is essentially the same as the false heat described in the Fire chapter. It can also be thought of as deficient Water of the Kidneys, which is unable to control Kidney Fire. Deficient Yin causes a *relative* excess of Yang: This means there are signs of heat, but they are not full or excessive (partial flushing, fevers only in the afternoon, etc.).

When the Water of the Kidneys is deficient, the other elements may present as follows:

EARTH ↑
may be excess and
overcontrolling Water

FIRE ↑
will be excess, further
consuming the body's Yin
(backing up into Water)

METAL ↓
may be deficient
and undernourishing
its child

WOOD ↑
will be excess, and draining
its mother

WATER
When the Water of
Water is the primary
imbalance (Kidney
Yin deficiency)

Ellen Z. came to acupuncture for treatment of symptoms associated with menopause. She complained of hot flashes, insomnia, night sweats, anxiety, and terrible mood swings, which made her alternately weepy, angry, and strangely euphoric.

Menopause often causes classic signs of deficient Yin, as this is a time when Yin's cooling and feminine qualities are being rapidly reduced. Hot flashes—heat in the upper body—are signs of rising Fire, which has no Water to control it. Insomnia and night sweats occur when

Yin is unable to contain Yang during the night, when it properly should do so. Anxiety and mood swings are signs of Shen, or Spirit, disturbance. These are caused by deficient Yin causing deficient blood in the Heart, which then fails to properly house the spirit.

Treatment for Ellen focused on building Kidney and Liver Yin, building Blood, and calming the spirit.

Kidney Yang Deficiency

Kidney Yang deficiency causes an apparent over-abundance of Yin, leading to conditions of coldness, water retention, and an overall lack of drive. The "Water excess" mentioned in later sections of this chapter does not refer to a true excess, but to Kidney Yang deficiency, the signs of which include:

* fatigue
* weakness
* cold limbs
* frequent urination
* edema/water retention
* low back ache or pain
* achy knees
* complaints that worsen in the morning
* diarrhea
* urgent bowel movements in the morning
* poor appetite

Creatively, Kidney Yang deficiency is the same as a Fire-element deficiency—it results in an inability

There were no atoms yet, let alone stars or galaxies: All was empty. We tend to think of it as a serene, hushed nothingness, an insubstantial, uneventful void, but it was in fact seething with all the pent-up energy of the primordial explosion.

—Trinh Xuan Thuan,
The Birth of the Universe: The Big Bang and After

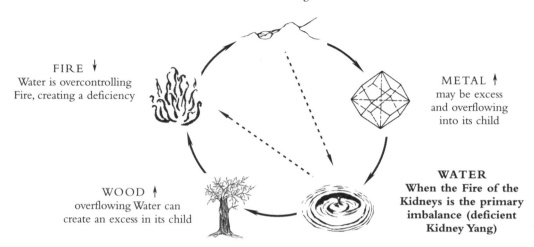

EARTH ↓
deficient Earth may be
undercontrolling Water

FIRE ↓
Water is overcontrolling
Fire, creating a deficiency

METAL ↑
may be excess
and overflowing
into its child

WOOD ↑
overflowing Water can
create an excess in its child

WATER
**When the Fire of the
Kidneys is the primary
imbalance (deficient
Kidney Yang)**

to follow through on ideas. One might have good ideas but will not have enough energy to begin a creative process.

When Yang deficiency becomes systemic, it often manifests in the Spleen and Heart as well, causing Earth and Fire deficiencies.

James G. came to acupuncture in February complaining of low back pain that ran all the way down to his knees. It bothered him especially in the early mornings, and when standing for long periods of time on a cold cement floor, which he often had to do in his job. James also complained of tiredness, and felt that he could never get enough sleep. His sleep was frustrating, too, because he usually had to wake up several times a night to urinate.

James's back and knee pain is a clear sign of Kidney dysfunction. The fact that it bothered him especially in the mornings, when Yang should properly be abundant, indicates deficient Yang. When he first showed up in February—the middle of winter—it was pretty clear that too much of Water element's cold was a main issue. Chronic sleepiness also indicates a lack of Kidney Fire, as does the frequent urination—particularly at night.

James's treatment was designed to warm the Fire of Kidneys.

Combined Kidney
Yin and Yang Deficiency

Because Yin and Yang create each other, a prolonged deficiency of either Yin or Yang will lead to a deficiency in the other as well. Kidney Yin and Kidney Yang can therefore be deficient at the same time with combined Yin- and Yang-deficient signs, like exhaustion and inability to sleep, or cold limbs, achy back and knees, and graying hair. Therefore, most remedies for Water deficiency include tonification of both Yin and Yang.

Manic-Depression: A Case of True Water Excess

While most traditions of acupuncture do not recognize any condition of Water excess, the emotional disease of manic depression does seem to involve excesses of both Kidney Yin and Kidney Yang—in alternating cycles. The depressive half of the cycle corresponds to a Kidney Yin excess, where one delves deeply in Water's eternal abyss, manifesting depression and a deep interiority that can verge on catatonia. When Kidney Yang is excessive, one flies euphorically into Fire's transcendent flames, exhibiting abundant activity, mania, creativity, movement, and Fire.

Since Yin and Yang create each other, excesses in one will tend to alternate cyclically with excesses in the other, resulting in the manic-depressive cycle known as bipolar disorder. The by-now-well-documented connection between manic-depression and supranormal creativity supports this conception of Water excess, wherein one suffers from an abundance of Water's creativity.

WATER AND ACUPUNCTURE

As with the other meridians, the Five Element points of the Kidney and Bladder meridians, located on the legs, are used to manipulate the dynamics of the Five Element cycle.

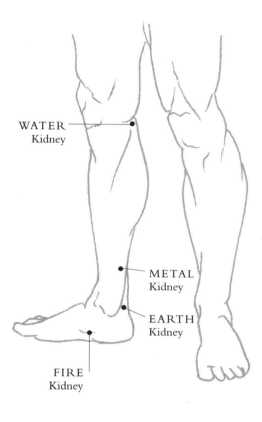

WATER
Kidney

METAL
Kidney

EARTH
Kidney

FIRE
Kidney

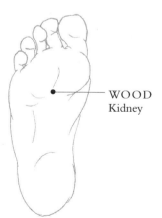

WOOD
Kidney

The Five Element Points on the
Kidney Meridian

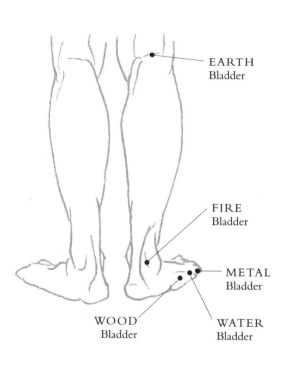

EARTH
Bladder

FIRE
Bladder

METAL
Bladder

WOOD
Bladder

WATER
Bladder

The Five Element Points on the
Bladder Meridian

The **Wood** points on the Water meridians influence the relationship between Water and its child in the Creation cycle. If an excess Wood element is draining its mother, for instance, Wood points can be dispersed. They can also be tonifed to encourage excess Water energy to move toward its child.

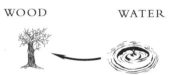

WOOD   WATER

The **Fire** points on Water meridians are often dispersed when Water is not controlling Fire.

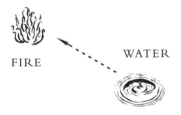

FIRE   WATER

The **Earth** points on Water meridians are likely to be used when Water is deficient due to Earth's overcontrol.

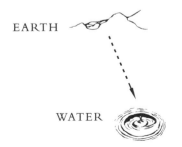

EARTH

WATER

The **Metal** points on Water meridians can be tonified to strengthen deficient Water through its mother, or during any other time when the relationship between Metal and Water needs to be adjusted.

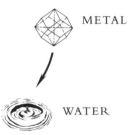

METAL

WATER

The **Water** points on Water meridians are good to use whenever Water energy is needed—to help control overactive Fire, for instance, or to nourish Wood.

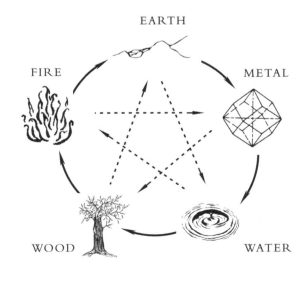

EARTH

FIRE   METAL

WOOD   WATER

WATER AND FOOD

The preparation, consumption, and digestion of food are some of our most basic activities, but they are not directly compatible with the Water phase, which requires tranquillity. Earth processes like eating and digesting cannot take place in a Water phase, nor can Water's rest take place during eating. However, food is still integral to the Water phase in a number of ways. As with the other elements, certain foods support Water and help to create it once they have been digested. Secondly, the Water element creates Essence (see QiGong section on page 194) partly from the foods we eat. In a sense, the Water element is the reason we eat in the first place: It represents the whole of our being, whose continuance requires appropriate nutrition.

Water's flavor: salty

Salty is a Yin flavor. It moves energy downward and inward, moistens dryness, softens hard lumps, stimulates appetite, and improves digestion. These are centering and "Earthy" qualities; Water, like the other elements, corresponds to a flavor that mimics its controlling element. Salty foods penetrate the Kidneys and Bladder, where they help to regulate water metabolism. Small amounts of salty foods can thus be included whenever the Water element is out of balance, although larger amounts will weaken it.

Salty foods include salt, seaweed, and soy sauce. In addition, barley and millet are grains that are considered both salty and sweet. Although there are fewer salty foods than any others, table salt is so overused in most diets that we hardly need other forms of it.* Salty herbs include oyster shell, kelp, and pumice.

Because salty foods exert an energy that controls Water, they are best eaten when Water is overactive—during times of fear or panic, for instance, or during Winter, when Water's cold needs to be controlled. It also helps to moisten certain dry conditions like constipation, and helps to draw toxins out of the body. Seaweeds like kelp and hijiki are best for this purpose.

Salt easily weakens the Kidneys and Bladder, however, disrupting water metabolism and leading to edema, urinary difficulties, and dampness conditions as well as other weaknesses of the Water element. In addition, a weakened Water element will be unable to control Fire, leading to hypertension and heart disease—conditions that Western medicine also recognizes as being aggravated by the overconsumption of salt.

Water's thermal nature: cool/cold

Just as Fire epitomizes the warming nature of foods, Water represents those foods that are cold or cooling. Cooling

---

* The table salt commonly used is a refined product that is not properly balanced and should not be eaten. Sea salt, soy sauce, and miso are more healthful ways to include salt in the diet.

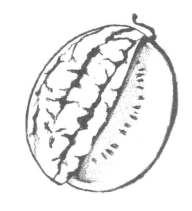

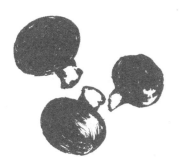

foods create quieter, slower, and more restful conditions in the body. They are best eaten when Water is deficient and needs to be strengthened—particularly during heat or Fire conditions that need Water to control them.

Some examples of cooling foods include apples, bananas, pears, watermelons, cantaloupes, tomatoes, citrus fruits, lettuce, radishes, cucumbers, celery, swiss chard, spinach, broccoli, cauliflower, corn, zucchini, soy milk, tofu, alfalfa sprouts, millet, barley, wheat and wheat products, amaranth, kelp and all seaweeds, algaes, yogurts, crabs, and clams.

Cooling foods should not be eating during cold or damp conditions (Water or Earth excesses), as they will aggravate those conditions.

Water's vegetables: seaweeds, fungi, and squashes

Water's vegetables and fruits grow in a suspended manner and tend to propagate horizontally, spreading outward like waves or ripples. Seaweeds grow in this manner and are also salty, which further strengthens their affinity with the Water element. Mushrooms and other fungi grow in wet, dark, and cool conditions, and propagate by the spread of spores. They, too, resonate strongly with the Water element. Squashes grow suspended from their vines, and also share an affinity with Water. All these foods can be eaten to tonify a deficient Water element and to cool Fire. They need to be avoided, however, in conditions of dampness and cold.

Water's fruits: melons and grapes

Water's fruits grow, like its vegetables, suspended from their stalks. Melons and grapes thus share Water's characteristics and can be eaten to cool the body, remove toxins, and control Fire. They should be avoided in conditions of cold, damp, and extreme Fire deficiency.

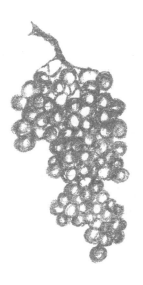

Water's colors: blue, black, and purple

Foods with blue, black, and purple coloring support the Kidneys and Bladder, cool the body, tonify Yin, and control Fire. Some examples of these foods include black beans, black sesame seeds, blueberries, blackberries, dark grapes, blue corn, eggplant, purple potatoes, and wild rice. Like other Water-tonifying foods, these should not be eaten with cold or damp conditions.

Tonifying Water Deficiency

A Water-deficiency diet is useful to cool the heat of summer, and for recovery from hot and/or feverish illnesses. One of the best ways to tonify Water deficiency is to drink plenty of water—filtered or spring water is best. Water deficiency can also be tonified with Water's fruits and vegetables, Water's colors, and very small amounts of salty foods in the diet. In addition, cooling foods and foods that tonify Metal can also help to tonify Water through its mother in the Creation cycle. Cooking methods that use a lot of water—like steaming, boiling, and poaching—are also helpful.

Controlling Water Excess: Food and Winter

Winter foods—or any foods eaten to control Water's excess—need to be warming and stabilizing to boost the Yang and Fire of the Kidneys. Salty and sweet flavors unify and descend energy, helping your body to accord with the winter season and internal cold conditions. Soups and stews as well as roasted meats and vegetables are good for these conditions, as are Water-element foods like beans and winter squash, and steamed winter greens like escarole and endive.

In general, meals should be larger, heartier, and cooked with methods that use higher heat for longer periods of time—baking, roasting, and frying. In addition, foods that tonify Earth, as described in the Earth chapter, will help to control excess Water, while Fire-tonifying and warming foods will help to combat winter's cold.

WATER AND QIGONG

The Water element is essential to the study of QiGong, as it creates and maintains Essence, one of QiGong's Three Treasures. Essence is the material "stuff" of which the universe is composed, as well as the spark of divinity that infills it. Often called "vitality," Essence is the ineffable something that distinguishes life from nonlife: the essence of existence. In many ways Essence is consistent with the Western understanding of soul; it is the material aspect of divinity.

WATER EXCESS RECIPE
Salmon Steaks with Sesame Seeds

5 salmon steaks

3 tsp. fresh lime juice

1 tsp. olive oil

2 tsp. soy sauce

2 tsp. sesame oil

1/2 tsp. grated fresh ginger

5 tbsp. black sesame seeds

1 tbsp. celery seeds

butter

1. Marinate steaks in lime juice, olive oil, soy sauce, sesame oil, and ginger. Let stand loosely covered for about an hour.

2. Preheat oven to 350°F.

3. Spread sesame seeds and celery seeds in a small pan. Toast them in the oven for 3 to 5 minutes until slightly brown. Do not burn. Shake or turn them midway through the toasting.

4. When the salmon is ready to cook, preheat the broiler.

5. Broil salmon until done, about 5 minutes per side.

6. Sprinkle the cooked salmon with the mixed toasted sesame and celery seeds. Serve with one or two pats of chilled butter.

In the universe, Essence is the light of the sun, moon, and stars. It is the existence of galaxies and the omnipresent underlayer of the Tao. On earth, Essence is the spark in all living things as well as the physical forms they take. Thus, bodies and branches, molecules and materials, are all composed of Essence.

In the body, Essence is both the flesh-and-blood body and the root of life within it. Like a battery cell, Essence stores potential, which is converted throughout our lives into energy. It also forms the substance of our bodies, and is responsible for growth and development, sexual secretions, and sexual activity. Essence carries our genetic and karmic blueprints, our will to live, and our desire to procreate; it is the source of our earthly existence.

Essence is partly inherited from our

parents and partly created from the purest aspects of food and air. It is stored in our Kidneys, and converted bit by bit into the Yin and Yang energies that power our bodies. When Essence is used up, however, life ends. Its regulation and preservation is therefore the root of longevity, which has historically been a prime focus of Taoist and Chinese medical traditions.

The ways to preserve and produce Essence are the sum total of all the healthy practices prescribed by Chinese Medicine:

* healthy eating habits—good foods and the care and protection of the Spleen as described in the Earth chapter
* good breathing habits as described in the Metal chapter
* healthy lifestyle habits—the balance of work and rest, the emotions, sexual activity, etc., as described in the Earth chapter
* meditation as described in the Fire chapter
* exercises as described in the Wood chapter

All these activities affect Essence both in its production and in its preservation. Proper eating habits, for example, use minimal amounts of stored Essence to help digest food properly. At the same time, they increase the amount of fresh Essence that can be extracted from the foods during digestion. Essence is thus preserved in two ways when our eating habits are well regulated. Improper eating habits, on the other hand, use inordinate amounts of stored Essence while inhibiting the organs' capacity to extract more.

Exercises preserve Essence by removing obstructions that drain it, and by creating a healthier body, which can then better extract fresh Essence from food and air. The external exercises described in the Wood chapter are practiced for this purpose. Internal exercises, however, are designed expressly for the regulation of Essence. Rather than contributing to health and longevity like the external practices, internal exercises involve spiritual training and the quest for enlightenment. They require physical as well as mental discipline, including meditation, breath work, and movement.

Although many of these practices

*Promoting Essence: The Jade Hop**
To Be Practiced Fully Naked

Stand upright with your feet shoulder-width apart or slightly wider. Raise the arms just above shoulder height alongside the body, and bend the elbows so that your hands face upward and toward each other just above your head. Relax your shoulders and straighten the back of your neck by tucking the chin in slightly. Hop up and down, rapidly but gently, for a minute or two or until you are winded. As you hop, curl and uncurl your fingers every two to three hops, making sure to relax them fully when you uncurl them.

This exercise will cause women's breasts, and men's testicles and penis, to bounce up and down. The exercise stimulates the flow of qi and Blood in the sexual organs and the endocrine glands that secrete hormones. It also stimulates Kidney Essence.

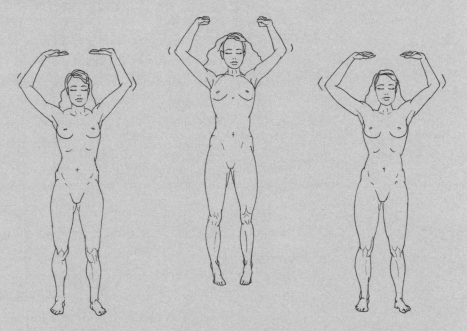

* Adapted from Daniel Reid, *The Complete Book of Chinese Health and Healing: Guarding the Three Treasures.*

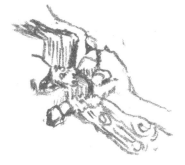

waterfall

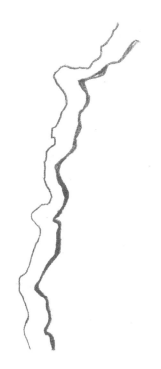

meandering river shape

are considered secret and sacred, some good books are available, in particular *The Brain/Marrow Washing Classic of Chuang Zu,* as translated by Yang Jwin-Ming, and Daniel P. Reid's *The Complete Book of Chinese Health and Healing: Guarding the Three Treasures.* The preceding "sexercise" from Reid's book is intended to build Essence through the creation of sexual secretions. It is not meant to be used for sexual activity but for the solitary meditative practice of building Essence.

WATER AND FENG SHUI

Water in Feng Shui occurs wherever there is water, the colors blue or black, darkness, coolness, and undulating or irregular surfaces. Although dark and cool spots are associated with Yin and therefore with the Water element, water in Feng Shui generally refers to watercourses—oceans, rivers, lakes, pools, and fountains. These are thought to bring health and prosperity to those who dwell nearby.

In classical Feng Shui, the natural flow of water is thought to be meandering and curvy; straight watercourses are considered to force too much qi along a specific path, which is harmful to whatever lies in that path. Water should move—not lie still, although water that moves too quickly is not good either. A lapping bay, a meandering river, or a bubbling pool or lake are all good sources of water to have near the home. Clear, healthy water attracts money, so that homes or businesses with a view of water are thought to be more propitious than ones without.

Water that embraces a dwelling on three sides (like a bay) is considered most fortuitous, while water that runs away from the home takes away the inhabitants' money.

In an urban landscape, roads and driveways can be considered as watercourses. The flow of traffic along them is similar to the flow of water. For this reason, a circular drive is considered more beneficial than a straight one, which channels traffic too directly toward the house. Straight roads are therefore problematic—they channel qi too quickly—and should not be directed toward a home or business.

The mountains that correspond to Water are irregular and undulating foothills, valleys, and ridges. Water buildings are those with irregular roofs—like tiles or thatch. In addition, architectural details like carvings and stonemasonry create a Watery surface.

Indoors, black and deep blues are the color of water. Water shapes are irregular or concave, like carpets, upholstery (because of their undulating surfaces), sinks and tubs, curtains, and tapestries. Carved surfaces also correspond to the Water element. Water materials are liquids—water and glass.

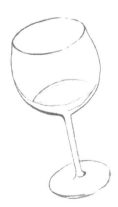

Tonifying Water Deficiency

To tonify Water deficiency, emphasize peace and stillness, and seek the wisdom of your inner voice. Wear black and blue colors, dim the lights, spend time sitting, sleeping, or meditating. The most important activity for Water deficiency is inactivity. Learn how to spend a day on the couch. Read or watch TV if you must, but try to spend a portion of your time doing nothing but reflecting. Try gazing into a fish tank or a deep bowl filled with water and letting your mind just float. Look at photographs or works of art to stimulate memories, reveries, and day-dreams. Take a bath, go for a swim, or listen to the ocean or a babbling brook. Sound—including music—is an important tool of the Water element, nourishing it through the ears, which are governed by the Kidneys.

A good way to get back in sync with a wounded Water element is to pay attention to your dreams. Keep a dream journal, and spend the first part of every day writing and thinking about the images in your dreams.

In addition, follow the instructions for tonifying Metal, and for reducing Earth.

Dispersing Water Excess

Water excess usually manifests as cold. Keep your body warm with clothing, hot drinks, hot water bottles, and exercise. Bring fire into your life to ward off cold. Light candles and incense. Keep rooms well lit. Eat warm and spicy foods. Counter Water's dark and stillness with bright colors, physical activity, and warmth. Drain Water excess by emphasizing Wood activities like exercise and writing or some other creative activity. Emphasize shape, form, and boundary in everything you do. Control Water excess by tonifying Earth as described in the Earth chapter. Contain Water's formlessness by focusing on form.

The Ba-Gua area that corresponds to Water is the north. It is also associated with career, and with the ears. To adjust a Water imbalance or to stimulate your career, try placing a fish tank or fountain along the north wall of a den or living room. A landscape painting that includes both water and mountains would be helpful as well. Alternatively, any Feng Shui standard cure—mirrors, plants, lights, etc.—can be used to rectify this Ba-Gua area.

The northeast corresponds to knowledge and self-cultivation. This is an ideal location for a desk or bookshelf, and can be further stimulated by mirrors, artwork, plants, or fountains.

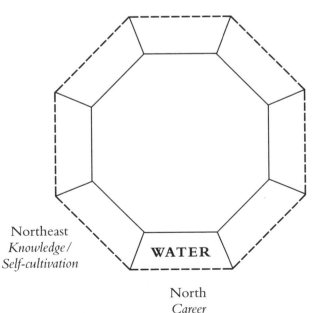

Northeast
Knowledge/
Self-cultivation

WATER

North
Career

As if it were the moment before the actual instant of creation, the last second before the awesome command: Let there be light!

I never feel so alone in the world, completely uprooted and at the same time completely soothed, so tense with yearning and at the same time, blissfully certain of ultimate fulfillment as in this hour before dawn and day.

—Felix Salten
Good Comrades

Winter Night

My bed is so
*   empty that I keep*
*   on waking up:*

As the cold
*   increases, the*
*   night wind begins*
*   to blow.*

It rustles the
*   curtains, making a*
*   noise like the sea;*

Oh that those were
*   waves which*
*   could carry me*
*   back to you!*

—Yang-ti

A well-balanced Water element allows us to move through the world with confidence and calm. It gives us a sense of strength and an awareness of our ability to handle even difficult situations. Water also provides for endless creativity and a love of relaxation and quietude. Healthy Water gives us a balanced perspective on our own struggles, and the ability to view the struggles of others with compassion.

Because of its deep interiority, the Water within us is easily drowned out by our busy lives and manifold obligations. When this happens, we lose touch with inner peace, wisdom, and our sense of knowing. We may feel exhausted, depressed, out of sync, or just plain irritable. This is a time to dive into our private oceans, to reacquaint ourselves with who we are and what we need. Only after we have taken this valuable time for ourselves can we begin to interact properly with the outside world. That interaction, when it comes out of consultation with our inner wisdom, leads to a dynamic and powerful Wood phase.

Brief Tenant

Out of the vast depths of time past,
    Man comes like a meteor's flash.

In myth, in dream, this living dust remembers

Chaos, the drift through endless night,
    the longing to cohere,

the shock, the winds, the vast light of creation.

Was it seven billion years ago this planet
    formed from the cosmic cloud?

How many billion when first life stirred in the seas?

Our blood is sea water: it remembers tides,
    the moon's pull.

In the hollow of the womb each of us
    is life evolving from the sea.

—Nancy Newhall
This Is the American Earth

I live my life in growing orbits
which move out over the things of the world.
Perhaps I can never achieve the last,
but that will be my attempt.

I am circling around God, around the ancient tower,
and I have been circling for a thousand years,
and I still don't know if I am a falcon, or a storm,
or a great song.

—Rainer Maria Rilke

CONCLUSION

Once you know what to look for, you'll discover the Five Element cycle everywhere you turn; in personalities, works of art, social movements, office politics, household objects, and more. Like ancient gods and goddesses, the elements appear in many manifestations. In your own life, you'll notice that you can be involved in hundreds of different cycles at the same time—in the Metal phase of a project, an Earth phase of life, and a Wood phase of a relationship with Earth symptoms at a Metal time of year. These interwoven cycles define the dynamic of our lives: many-layered, interconnected, and perpetually in motion.

With so many different aspects, the Five Elements can be approached on many levels. In one sense, the cycle brings insight to your daily experience. It suggests that you can wade through a period of Metal's grief by cleaning house, for instance, teaching this as an appropriate activity at such a time. Or it helps you recognize that your Wood element is sensitive when allergies flare up, so that you can make a concerted effort to not let anger get the best of you. Riding the tides of the Five Element cycle in this way helps you minimize stress by knowing what to emphasize and what to play down on a day-to-day basis.

On another level, you can use the Five Element cycle to make conscious changes in your life and health. You can pick an element that you feel particular kinship with, or choose an element that corresponds to a problem you're currently facing—Wood for irritability, for instance, or Water simply because it intrigues you. Determine whether that element tends toward deficiency or excess in you, then see if you can create change in that imbalance by following the suggestions in this book. Alter your eating habits, shift a few things around the house, change your exercise pattern, etc., according to the deficiency or excess you discover.

You may not notice until things start to change that the element you picked was out of balance in many areas of your life. You may find emotional symptoms where you'd recognized only physical ones, or environmental imbalances in what you'd thought was a personality conflict in your office. Amazingly, the simplest modifications in your habits can cause shifts to occur in feelings, relationships, symptoms, and behaviors that you hadn't even considered as being related to your main concern. You will find yourself healing in surprising and welcome ways, and learning about connection by experiencing it directly.

While Chinese culture is not the only one to have developed a system of medicine that interlocks with nature, it has done so with breathtaking detail. In defining the ways our bodies reflect these forces of the universe, the Five Element system declares that the planet and its creatures are made of the same stuff. We suffer the same illnesses, and will heal from the same cures: We are *that* closely intertwined. Perhaps the greatest gift of the Five Element cycle is this sense of intimacy it creates between ourselves and the rest of the universe. Indeed, it is a wonder to recognize that bird, flower, neighbor, planet, solar system, and you and I are all dancing the same primal dance. It is an echo of the music of creation, the definition of wholeness, and the goal of every healing.

In framing our private healing journeys this way, as holographic parts of a larger whole, we get a glimpse of what may be our proper place in the universe—both as individuals and as a species. Every illness we face challenges us to rediscover that place—the harmony within the whole. It is what healing is, and what medicine should strive for.

May God and the Goddess bless you on the journey, and may you find love and harmony in all things.

REFERENCES

Beinfield, Harriet, and Efrem Korngold. *Between Heaven and Earth: A Guide to Chinese Medicine.* New York: Ballantine Books, 1991.

Biedermann, Hans. *Dictionary of Symbolism.* New York: Penguin Books, 1992.

Bogdanovich, Peter (editor). *The White Goddess Engagement Diary 1997.* Woodstock, N.Y.: The Overlook Press.

Breslow, Arieh Lev. *Beyond the Closed Door: Chinese Culture and the Creation of T'ai Chi Ch'uan.* Jerusalem: The Almond Blossom Press, 1995.

Caso, Alfonso. *The Aztecs: People of the Sun.* Lowell Dunham, trans. Norman, Okla.: University of Oklahoma Press, 1958.

Chan Wing-Tsit. *A Source Book in Chinese Philosophy.* Princeton, N.J.: Princeton University Press, 1963.

Cheng Xinnong, ed. *Chinese Acupuncture and Moxibustion.* Beijing: Foreign Languages Press, 1987.

Cohen, Kenneth S. *The Way of QiGong: The Art and Science of Chinese Energy Healing.* New York: Ballantine Books, 1997.

Connelly, Dianne. *Traditional Acupuncture: The Law of the Five Elements.* Columbia, Md.: The Center for Traditional Acupuncture, 1975.

Cowan, Eliot. *Plant Spirit Medicine.* Newburg, Ore.: Swan Raven & Co., 1995.

Eitel, Ernest J. *Feng-Shui: The Science of Sacred Landscape in Old China.* Bonsall, Cal.: Synergetic Press, Inc., 1993.

Ellis, Andrew, Nigel Wiseman, and Ken Boss. *Fundamentals of Chinese Acupuncture.* Brookline, Mass.: Paradigm Publications, 1991.

Four Winds Development Project. *The Sacred Tree.* Twin Lakes, Wis.: Lotus Light Publications, 1989.

Fung Yu-Lan. *A History of Chinese Philosophy, Vol. I & II.* Derk Bodde, trans. Princeton, N.J.: Princeton University Press, 1983.

Gordon, Stuart. *The Encyclopedia of Myths and Legends.* London: Headline Book Publishing, 1993.

Guth, Alan, and Paul Steinhardt. "The Inflationary Universe," *The New Physics,* Paul Davies, ed. New York: Cambridge University Press, 1989.

Haas, Elson M. *Staying Healthy with the Seasons*. Berkeley, Cal.: Celestial Arts, 1981.

Hammer, Leon. *Dragon Rises, Red Bird Flies: Psychology and Chinese Medicine*. Barrytown, N.Y.: Station Hill Press, 1990.

Hawking, Stephen, "The Edge of Spacetime," *The New Physics*, Paul Davies, ed. New York: Cambridge University Press, 1989.

Heinberg, Richard. *Celebrate the Solstice*. Wheaton, Ill.: Quest Books, 1993.

Jarrett, Lonny S. "Chinese Medicine and the Betrayal of Intimacy: The Theory and Treatment of Abuse, Incest, Rape and Divorce with Acupuncture and Herbs—Part I." *American Journal of Acupuncture,* Vol. 23, No. 1, 1995.

Kaptchuk, Ted J. *The Web That Has No Weaver: Understanding Chinese Medicine*. New York: Congdon & Weed, Inc., 1983.

Lauterbach, Robert. *The World of Geology: The Earth Then and Now*. A.C. Bishop and E. Launert, trans.

German Democratic Republic: Edition Leipzig, 1983.

Lip, Evelyn. *Feng Shui: A Layman's Guide*. Torrance: Heian International, Inc., 1979.

Liu, Jilin, and Gordon Peck, eds. *Chinese Dietary Therapy*. New York: Churchill Livingstone, 1995.

Logan, William Bryant. *Dirt, the Ecstatic Skin of the Earth*. New York: Riverhead Books, 1995.

Maciocia, Giovanni. *The Foundations of Chinese Medicine*. New York: Churchill Livingstone, 1989.

Matsumoto, Kiiko, and Stephen Birch. *Five Elements and Ten Stems*. Brookline, Mass.: Paradigm Publications, 1993.

Ni, Maoshing (translator). *The Yellow Emperor's Classic of Internal Medicine*. Boston, Mass.: Shambhala Publications, Inc., 1995.

Ni, Maoshing, and Cathy McNease. *The Tao of Nutrition*. Santa Monica: Seven Star Communications Group, Inc., 1987.

Pitchford, Paul. *Healing with Whole Foods: Oriental Traditions and Modern Nutrition*, Rev. Ed. Berkeley: North Atlantic Books, 1993.

Reid, Daniel. *The Complete Book of Chinese Health & Healing.* Boston, Mass.: Shambhala Publications, Inc., 1995.

Rossbach, Sarah. *Interior Design with Feng Shui.* New York: E. P. Dutton, 1987.

Rossbach, Sarah, and Lin Yun. *Living Color: Master Lin Yun's Guide to Feng Shui and the Art of Color.* New York: Kodansha America, 1994.

Schipper, Kristofer. *The Taoist Body.* Berkeley and Los Angeles: The University of California Press, 1993.

Skinner, Stephen. *The Living Earth Manual of Feng-Shui: Chinese Geomancy.* New York: Penguin, 1982.

Thuan, Trinh Xuan. *The Birth of the Universe: The Big Bang and After.* New York: Harry N. Abrams, Inc., 1993.

Unschuld, Paul U. *Medicine in China: A History of Ideas.* Berkeley and Los Angeles: University of California Press, 1985.

Waley, Arthur. *Translations from the Chinese.* New York: Alfred A. Knopf, 1919, 1941.

Walker, Barbara G. *Woman's Dictionary of Symbols and Sacred Objects.* New York: HarperCollins Publishers, Inc., 1988.

Walker, Barbara G. *Woman's Encyclopedia of Myths and Secrects.* New York: HarperCollins Publishers, Inc., 1983.

Wilhelm, Richard and Cary F. Baynes, trans. *The I-Ching or Book of Changes.* Princeton, N.J.: Princeton University Press, 1977.

Yang Jwing-Ming. *The Root of Chinese Chi Kung: The Secrets of Chi Kung Training.* Jamaica Plain, Mass.: YMAA Publication Center, 1995.

Yuen, Jeffrey. Notes from September 1993 lecture at the Tri-State Institute of Traditional Chinese Acupuncture.

If you would like to find a licensed or certified acupuncturist or herbalist in your area, call the National Commission for the Certification of Acupuncture and Oriental Medicine at 1-202-232-1404.

INDEX

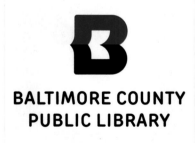